evaluating
clinical
research

Bengt D. Furberg and Curt D. Furberg

evaluating
clinical
research

All that glitters is not gold

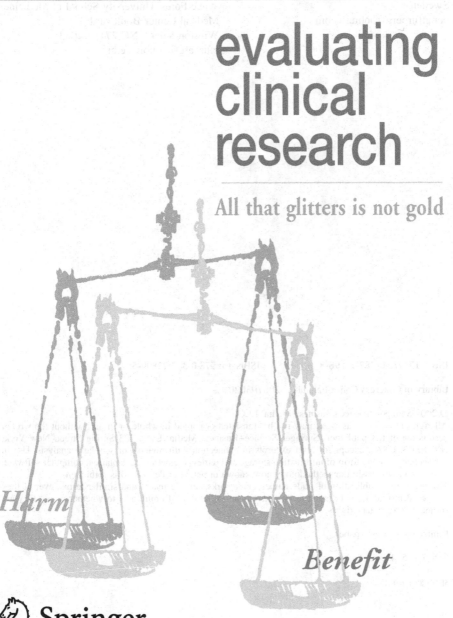

Harm

Benefit

Springer

Bengt D. Furberg, MD, PhD
Associate Professor
S-434 46 Kungsbacka
Sweden
bengtfurberg@hotmail.com

Curt D. Furberg, MD, PhD
Professor
Division of Public Health Sciences
Wake Forest University School of Medicine
Medical Center Boulevard
Winston-Salem, NC 27157-1063
cfurberg@wfubmc.edu

ISBN-13: 978-0-387-72898-8   e-ISBN-13: 978-0-387-72899-5

Library of Congress Control Number: 2007930204

Printed on acid-free paper.

9 8 7 6 5 4 3 2 1

springer.com

Contents

Chapter 1

What is the purpose of this book?

This edition updates and expands the first edition of this text, released in 1994. Its purpose is unchanged — to guide clinicians and others in the health care field as well as employees in companies manufacturing drugs, devices and other medical products. Our hope is that the advice will assist the reader in understanding the strengths and weaknesses of clinical studies and in distinguishing patient-important and methodologically sound studies from those, which are limited by design, operational constraints and interpretation.

Clinical trials are used to evaluate drugs, surgical procedures, medical devices, dietary counseling, physiotherapy and other potential interventions. Increasingly, we rely on the results of these trials to guide the decision on whether to allow a new treatment to become part of established medical practice. Most of the examples in this book are from actual drug trials.

Selecting the safest and the most effective therapy is the goal of all patient care. This goes back to the Oath of Hippocrates and the commitment *primum non nocere* (first do no harm). The selection of optimal treatments also has

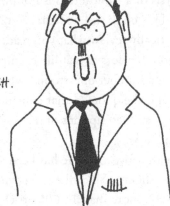

— MY NICHE IN SCIENCE IS TO FIND ERRORS IN OTHER PEOPLE'S RESEARCH.

important social implications, as there is now a greater focus on cost-benefit considerations in medicine. Patients assume health care professionals know about the most up-to-date and favorable treatments, so it is important that all physicians possess the necessary skills to review critically scientific publications, especially those about medications that they might prescribe to their patients.

However, most health care professionals have received little training either in research methodology or in the critical appraisal of clinical trial results. Continuing medical education programs certainly help to fill some of this knowledge gap, and there are several excellent texts on clinical trial issues.[1-3] However, these typically target researchers who design and analyze their own studies rather than practicing clinicians. Available texts are often lengthy and may concentrate on statistical and methodological issues that are of little direct interest to those who primarily deliver patient care.

In this book, we focus on patient-important issues. There is no mention of phase I trials, which provide an initial assessment of agents that have shown promise in animal models. We also exclude a discussion of phase II trials, which consider drug dosing, safety and early clinical evidence of therapeutic potential in a small number of patients. The findings of phase I and II trials form the basis of the decision to proceed to larger phase III trials, which evaluate the balance of benefit-to-harm in a more generalized patient population.

Biostatistics is a fundamental part of clinical research. The planning, design and analysis of a clinical trial is not possible without special knowledge of biostatistics. This book will not turn you into a statistical expert, but it will enable you to critically review what you read. There are no statistical formulas or technical jargon, but lots of real-life examples drawn from clinical research. We have included a number of cartoons, which are sometimes provocative. The Key Points and the quotes[4,5] that conclude each chapter emphasize the take-home messages. Descriptions of selected terms are presented in the Glossary (Appendix A).

Over the past 15 years, there has been a shift from opinion-based to evidence-based medicine. Since the term evidence-based medicine was introduced in 1992, more than 15,000 articles and books have been published on this topic. Informative and independent reviews or research studies covering a broad array of medical disciplines are available, for example, through the Cochrane Collaboration and through other web-based sources as discussed in Chapter 25. These reviews are time-saving for the busy professional because they usually distill a lot of information from a number of sources. Nonetheless, there is no substitute for reviewing scientific evidence personally to fully understand the benefit–to-harm balance of a specific intervention.

"All that glisters is not gold"
(W. Shakespeare in "The Merchant of Venice")

Why is benefit-to-harm balance essential to treatment decisions?

The 1962 amendments to the U.S. Federal Food, Drug and Cosmetic Act require that for a new drug to be approved for marketing, there needs to be substantial evidence of both safety and efficacy when the drug is prescribed for its intended indication(s). In other words, a drug has to have beneficial effects that outweigh any potential harm; it has to have what is known as a favorable, or positive, benefit-to-harm balance. This is also true of other types of interventions such as medical devices and diagnostic procedures.

- WEIGHING BENEFIT VERSUS HARM REQUIRES A BALANCED SCALE.
- WHERE CAN I GET ONE?

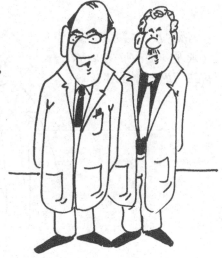

What are the goals of treatment?

In general, there are three main goals of treating a patient:
- to make the patient feel better
- to reduce the risk of future disease complications
- to improve survival

There are those who include a fourth goal, "economic benefit," both to the patient and to society, e.g., returning to work, supporting family, paying taxes, reducing future demands on the healthcare system. Our view is that economic benefit represents a natural consequence of reaching one or more of the three main goals.

Although a particular treatment might be effective, it may not necessarily achieve all three goals. A painkiller or a drug for nausea might instantly improve a patient's well-being, but it would not be expected to bring any long-term benefit. In contrast, a drug to treat hypertension may reduce the long-term risks of cardiovascular complications and premature death without any tangible benefit to the patient, since most people with high blood pressure are asymptomatic. Some interventions may achieve all three goals. Effective antibiotic treatment of acute bacterial meningitis relieves symptoms, reduces the risk of neurologic complications, and decreases short-term mortality.

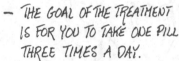

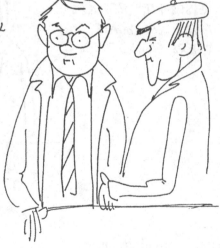

How is the benefit of a treatment documented?

Controlled clinical trials designed to determine whether a therapy prolongs life or reduces the risks of major non-fatal complications typically require thousands of study subjects treated for years. Diseases with very high complication rates or high mortality such as subarachnoidal hemorrhage or

pancreatic cancer are the exception. Except in these instances, evaluating whether a treatment reduces complications or improves survival takes a lot of time and is very costly. To document that a treatment provides symptomatic relief is less time-consuming and cheaper. For many chronic conditions, symptomatic improvement rather than clinical cure may be the most realistic goal and most prescription drugs are given with this intention. Difficulties associated with the assessment of symptoms are discussed in Chapter 11.

It is the responsibility of the manufacturer to document the value of a new product. Since a considerable investment of time and resources is needed to evaluate the effect of any treatment on survival or on the risks of disease complications, it is not surprising that there has been a lot of interest in biologic markers, or so-called surrogate endpoints. Evaluating the effect of various treatments on factors associated with the risk of disease, such as elevation of LDL cholesterol, systolic blood pressure and HbA_{1C}, has paid off handsomely for manufacturers. Several widely prescribed drugs have been approved for marketing based on a favorable effect on risk factors rather than definitive evidence of a true health benefit to patients. The value of these markers and the difficulties in drawing conclusions about their clinical utility based on treatment-induced changes are discussed in Chapters 13 and 19, respectively.

How is the harm of a treatment documented?
No treatment is free of adverse effects or harm. Any treatment decision ought to be based on weighing the likely favorable effects against the unfavorable ones.

A common complaint of patients is that a prescribed medication made him/her feel worse. The problem can range from something simple such as dryness of the mouth to serious adverse events that may require the treatment to be stopped. Even simple adverse effects can be very distressing for the patient, thereby reducing compliance. Adverse effects with a gradual onset are the most difficult to detect because the patient may not attribute them immediately to the treatment. Assessment of the patient's quality-of-life may sometimes help to detect modest changes in well-being due to the effects of a medication.

Occasionally, drugs may have serious adverse effects such as allergic reactions, hepatitis, cardiac arrhythmias and gastric ulcer. Despite this, attributing an adverse event to a specific treatment can sometimes be difficult, particularly when the event is rare, unexpected, or appears a long time after the start of treatment. It can also be difficult to recognize an adverse effect when it may occur as part of the natural history of the underlying condition. These challenges are discussed in Chapter 4.

Limited clinical experience with a drug when it is first marketed may result in it having a more "favorable" benefit-to-harm balance than it deserves. It has been estimated that as many as half of all new drugs have at least one serious adverse effect that is unknown at the time of drug approval.

Many drugs are metabolized in the liver and an emerging area of concern is the possibility of drug-drug interactions. Toxicity may occur when one drug inhibits the metabolism of another drug, or when two drugs compete for the same metabolic pathway. Of all the potential interactions, only those between

- DOC, ANY RISK OF SIDE
  EFFECTS WITH THIS DRUG?
- NONE THAT YOU DON'T
  ALREADY HAVE.

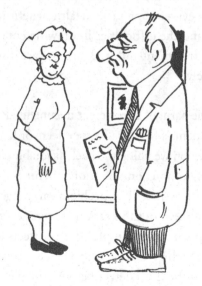

the most commonly prescribed drugs can be evaluated prior to marketing. In 1997, the FDA approved mibefradil (Posicor) for marketing in the U.S. The product was withdrawn within one year, after multiple serious drug interactions were documented, the most important one with simvastatin (Zocor).

There may also be other harmful effects of drugs that are less obvious. For example, some hormones, antibiotics and medications with prolonged half-lives may contribute to ecologic problems.

The high cost of an intervention may also be considered an adverse factor to patients and to society. Newer drugs with only incremental benefit are often much more expensive than older generic agents. "Patient labeling" can be an adverse effect of drug treatment itself. It has been reported that otherwise asymptomatic subjects who are placed on antihypertensive treatment develop various symptoms, since taking their medication serves as a reminder that they are not healthy.

Why off-label use of drug should be avoided?

One purpose of the important regulatory process of drug approval is to assure the public that approved drugs are both safe and efficacious. Randomized clinical trials represent essential tools in drug evaluation and they are usually required for regulatory approval. Manufacturers are only permitted to market drugs to health care providers and the public for the approved indication.

In contrast to the drug approval process, the practice of medicine is not regulated, so healthcare professionals can prescribe drugs for unapproved uses if they believe this is in the best interests of the patient. The pharmaceutical industry takes advantage of this through "indirect" marketing of its drugs for unapproved indications. This so-called "off-label" use is common. A study of 160 commonly prescribed drugs used among office-based physicians revealed that 21% of prescriptions were off-label.[2] There was little or no scientific support for most of these uses.

Limited evidence of safety and efficacy, including dosing, exposes patients to unnecessary risks. The direct risk is that the off-label use of the drug is ineffective, or harmful, or maybe both. The indirect risk is that proven alternative treatments, should they exist, may be denied. Since off-label use of drugs is not evidence-based, it is generally to be discouraged. An exception may be in oncology, where it would be difficult to evaluate a chemotherapy agent in all tumor types and stages of disease prior to marketing.

In recent years, the government has attempted to regulate off-label promotion in response to subtle efforts by industry to conceal direct incentive payments to clinicians, questionable consultant contracts, and all-expense paid 'educational' trips. The alleged deceptive "off-label" marketing of gabapentin (Neurontin) was settled for $468 million.[1] A more recent example is human growth hormone, which was never approved either to spur growth in children who were not hormone-deficient, or to slow the aging process in adults. Yet it has been widely prescribed for both indications.

Key Points

- The value of a medical intervention is determined by its benefit-to-harm balance.
- This balance may vary among patients with the same diagnosis.
- Major treatment benefits range from symptomatic relief to prevention of disease complications to improved survival.
- Safety information is often limited when a new intervention is introduced.
- Early assessments of the benefit-to-harm balance tend to be overly optimistic.

"There are two sides to a coin"

Chapter 3

What are the strengths of randomized controlled clinical trials?

The term "clinical trial" has many definitions.[1] A feature that is common to all definitions is that a clinical trial is always *prospective*, that is the study subjects are followed forward in time. There is also general agreement that the purpose of a clinical trial is to evaluate one or more *interventions* and to compare it/them with another treatment, a *control*. Although the word "clinical" limits the term to studies of humans, the same general methodology can easily be applied to studies of animals and plants. Clinical trials of drugs are often *randomized*, but randomization is not required for classifying a clinical study as a clinical trial. This is also true for *blinding*, or masking, which is a feature of many clinical trials of drugs. The terms randomization and masking/blinding are discussed below as well as in Chapters 9 and 10.

Among research methodologies, randomized, blinded, controlled clinical trials typically rank very high in terms of reliability for evaluating treatments.[6] At the top of the ranking are meta-analyses of clinical trials.

What are the advantages of being prospective?

The prospective nature of clinical trials has many advantages. Before starting a clinical trial, a study protocol must be written and approved. This document specifies exactly how the trial will be conducted. It defines the study objectives and states one of these as the primary objective. The protocol must be approved by an Institutional Review Board (IRB) and, if evaluating an investigational drug, by regulatory agencies as well. This requirement serves as a safeguard against clinical trials with inappropriate designs that do not address the study objectives or that may expose study subjects to harm that is out of proportion to any expected benefit. Hypotheses must be specified beforehand to provide protection against post-hoc "hypotheses" that are formulated to fit the observed results. Readers of published articles are at a disadvantage since they rarely have access to study protocols and must rely on the trial investigators, regulatory agencies, or IRBs to protect trial integrity and adherence to the study requirements.

The prospective nature of a trial also has the advantage of giving the investigators control over the data collection. Retrospective studies are limited to old data, that is, information previously collected by others often for a very different purpose. Consequently, data in retrospective studies may be incomplete and of varying quality. A prospective study gives the investigator the opportunity to decide exactly what information to collect, as well as when and how to record it.

Further, prospective data collection enhances quality and allows monitoring of this process according to Guidance for Industry — Good Clinical Practice.[2] Data quality can also be improved through internal quality control procedures overseen by the trial sponsor and through inspections conducted by regulatory agencies. Retrospective studies lack all these measures to ensure data quality and integrity.

What is the difference between an intervention in a clinical trial and in an observational study?

The purpose of a clinical trial is to evaluate one or more interventions or a diagnostic procedure. The important distinction is that in a clinical trial the intervention is initiated by the investigator, while it is started by someone else in an observational study. Thus, clinical trials are "experimental," while observational studies are "non-experimental." A clinical trial has the advantage that the intervention follows a written protocol with defined patient inclusion and exclusion criteria that detail the precise characteristics of the enrolled study population. Drug dosing, dose adjustments, permitted concomitant medications, etc. are all predetermined. Also, a prospective trial allows for randomization, which means that the study groups are more likely to be comparable.

Why is a control group so important?

The major goals of medical treatment are to reduce or eliminate the symptoms and signs of a disease, to slow or halt disease progression, or to prevent specific complications, including premature death. The natural history of most diseases is unpredictable in individual patients. Several acute conditions such as the common cold are self-limiting; other diseases such as multiple sclerosis are often intermittent with unpredictable remissions. The time course of many chronic conditions is highly variable and the risk of complications of degenerative conditions such as atherosclerosis is unpredictable, although one can differentiate between low- and high-risk subjects. Consequently, distinguishing between real treatment effects and the natural course of a disease can be a major challenge. By using comparable groups of study subjects in a clinical trial, one receiving the new treatment and the other not, we are able to make a good estimate of both favorable and unfavorable treatment effects.

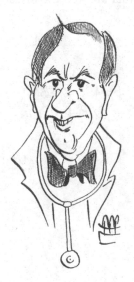

— IT'S EASIER FOR A NEW DRUG TO LOOK GOOD WHEN COMPARED TO NOTHING.

The increased attention given to subjects in a research project may influence study findings. This observation dates back to the 1920s. Employees of Hawthorne Works of the Western Electric Company in Chicago agreed to participate in a study designed to evaluate the effect of light levels on work performance.[5] Surprisingly, the work performance increased, regardless of whether the level of light at the workplace was increased, kept constant, or decreased. The special attention given to the workers who participated in the study explains the improvement in overall performance. This so-called *Hawthorne effect* refers to the tendency of people to alter their behavior when they are subject to special attention in a research setting. The use of a control group, especially in masked trials, "distributes" the Hawthorne effect on the trial findings evenly between the study groups.

What are the major advantages of randomization?

Randomization means that the allocation of subjects to one study group or another is determined by chance alone. To protect the integrity of the trial, it is critical that neither the investigator nor the study subject be involved in deciding to which group the subject is assigned. Experience has shown troubling imbalances between study groups in trials that allowed the investigator to control the allocation of subjects.

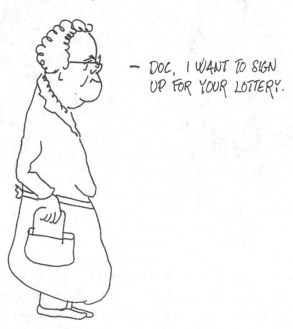

Tampering with the randomization process has been known to occur. Staff at one clinic in a large multicenter trial[3] opened the sealed randomization envelopes and arranged the assignments to Special Care or Usual Care to fit their own preferences.

Although proper randomization protects against bias in the allocation of subjects to the study groups, it does not guarantee that all groups at baseline are evenly matched for all known and unknown risk factors. Thus, randomization eliminates the systematic differences between study groups, but it cannot rule out some group differences due to chance. Nonetheless, randomization is one of the most important advantages that clinical trials have over observational studies, as discussed in Chapter 9.

Why is blinding/masking so important?

It is highly desirable that during the conduct of a clinical trial, study subjects and investigators, both of whom are in a position to influence reported benefits and adverse effects, are unaware of the allocated treatment. A well-executed double-blind design protects against "*ascertainment biases*" by blinding both parties to the assigned treatment. The terms blinding and masking are used interchangeably.

The potential problem is that investigators and study subjects involved in clinical studies often have pre-conceived hopes and expectations regarding the study outcome. This could influence the trial findings, since most methods to assess benefits and harm rely to some extent on subjective judgment. Thus, knowledge of group assignment may consciously or unconsciously influence the evaluation of treatment effects. This has been reported many times in the literature.

A classic illustration is a placebo-controlled vitamin C trial for the prevention and treatment of the common cold that was conducted among employees at the National Institutes of Health.[4] Many of the enrollees could not resist the temptation to analyze the content of their blinded study medications. Among the participants who did not break the blind, the mean duration of colds was similar in the two groups. In contrast, participants who knew they were taking vitamin C reported shorter cold durations than those who knew they took placebo!

Blinding is another major advantage of clinical trials compared to observational studies. Types and methods of blinding are discussed in Chapter 10.

Key Points
- The randomized, controlled, double-blind clinical trial is the "gold standard" for assessing treatment effects.
- The prospective nature of trials allows for better control over the completeness and quality of data collection.
- The use of a control group tends to compensate for non-treatment-related changes in disease status.
- Regulatory agencies usually require randomized clinical trials for drug approval.

"There is nothing like leather"

Chapter 4

What are the weaknesses of randomized controlled clinical trials?

The previous chapter concluded that randomized controlled clinical trials are the gold standard for evaluating the efficacy of medical interventions. However, the value of a treatment is not determined solely by its efficacy or benefit. It is also affected by adverse events, or harm, associated with its use. We should not forget that all clinical trials have an inherent weakness related to the assessment of safety.[6] To get a complete picture of the balance between benefit and harm of an intervention, safety information may need to be garnered from other sources such as non-experimental (observational) studies. In this chapter, we review important weaknesses of clinical trials related to safety — the detection of rare, late and unexpected adverse events.

Why are clinical trials unreliable for the detection of *rare* adverse events?

When a new pharmaceutical agent is approved for marketing, approximately 1,000 to 5,000 patients have typically been exposed to it. This number is adequate to determine the frequency of common, predictable, and easily recognized adverse effects. However, the likelihood of detecting rare adverse effects is small in clinical trials. This becomes more of an issue if the rare event is serious. Approximately 3,000 patients are required to detect a single case with 95% probability if its true incidence is one in 1,000; a total of 6,500 patients are needed to detect three cases. For very rare adverse effects with a true incidence of one in 10,000, at least 30,000 patients will have to be treated to detect one case. In order to detect three cases with 95% probability, 65,000 patients are required. These numbers illustrate why adverse effects with an incidence of one in 1,000 or less are very seldom detected in clinical trials. More commonly, these rare occurrences are discovered through case reports published as Letters to the Editor[8] or via reports of adverse events filed with regulatory agencies. Even then, the association of a particular adverse effect with a specific drug may only be made after there have been a cluster of cases reported. Clinical trials cannot be relied upon to detect rare adverse events.

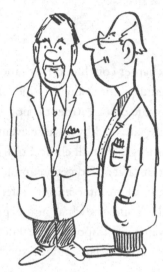

— WHY DO WE MISS
THE SIDE EFFECTS ?
— BECAUSE WE DON'T
LOOK FOR THEM.

Why are clinical trials unreliable for the detection of *late* adverse effects?

When a new compound intended for chronic or life-long use is introduced into the market, approximately a few hundred patients will have been treated for one year or longer. If the agent is an inhaled steroid for treatment of asthma, a lipid-lowering statin, or an antihypertensive drug, one can assume that the medications will be prescribed for longer than one year, maybe even for decades. Thus, one could legitimately question whether the one-year experience with the compound is adequate to predict drug safety over 5, 10, or up to 30 years. Many serious adverse events may take several years to become apparent. For example, it may take more than a decade of tobacco use to cause lung cancer. A safety profile based on limited drug exposure is inadequate and can be very misleading.

Several short-term studies of high doses of inhaled steroids have shown alterations in markers of bone metabolism. Leading scientists have concluded that these changes might lead to reduced bone density or osteoporosis, if steroids are used regularly over several years. A clinical trial designed to determine the risk of osteoporosis, or better yet the risk of bone fractures, would probably require a duration of 10 to 20 years. The comparison group could not be given steroids for this entire period and, additionally, controlling for confounding factors such as smoking, exercise and the use of estrogens would be a challenge. Realistically, it would be impossible to conduct such a trial. Few trials last more than four to five years. In summary, most clinical trials are not suitable for detection of adverse events that occur many years after initiation of treatment.

Why clinical trials have a limited value for detection of *unexpected* adverse events?

Many adverse effects of drugs are unexpected. For this reason, it may take several years before the occurrence of an adverse event is recognized and attributed to a specific medication. Terfenadine (Teldanex) had been on the market for more than a decade prior to the detection of a serious interaction with erythromycin or grapefruit juice that could cause a fatal arrhythmia.[1] Phenylpropanolamine (PPA) had been marketed even longer before there was a signal that it might cause intracranial hemorrhage.[5] Although these adverse effects are rare, they shift the balance between benefit and harm in an unfavorable direction, since the indications for these agents are not for life-threatening conditions, and there are effective and safe treatment alternatives.

Even very obvious adverse effects may be difficult to recognize if they are truly unexpected. Today we know that as many as 15-20% of users of ACE inhibitors develop dry cough, but it took several years after marketing of these drugs to establish this link. Why would anyone expect a potent class of drugs used for treatment of hypertension and congestive heart failure to cause cough?

Dexfenfluramine (Redux) was approved by the FDA as a promising drug for the treatment of obesity. However, bad news soon surfaced. The first cases of heart valve abnormalities were observed a year later, primarily in subjects exposed to the combination of fenfluramine and phentermine or "fen-phen."

Following the publication of a large case series[3] and reports to the FDA from several obesity clinics, dexfenfluramine was withdrawn from the market. The clinical experience suggested that use of dexfenfluramine for six months or longer caused an unknown type of valvulopathy in a small but significant proportion of subjects. It is notable that the clinical trial experience prior to drug approval, which included 1,000 subjects treated for one year, did not raise any suspicion about drug-induced valvular disease. How could this problem have been anticipated? It is no surprise that echocardiography was not a routine procedure in the clinical trials.

Vigabatrin (Sabrilex) is prescribed for the prevention of seizures in patients with epilepsy. By inhibiting so-called GAMA transaminase, the drug causes an increase of GABA, an important neurotransmitter in brain tissue. Following regulatory approval, it was reported in a European Union investigation that the drug caused visual field defects in as many as one-third of its users.[7] The unexpected adverse events were not reported during the pre-marketing clinical trials.

These examples illustrate that clinical trials of relatively large patient groups can fail to detect unexpected but potentially serious adverse effects. They are especially difficult to detect, if special examinations or procedures are required. The real answer can only come from asking the right question. The typical clinical trial is not a good source for detecting unexpected adverse drug effects.

— IT AIN'T EASY TO FIND THE RIGHT ANSWER WHEN YOU DON'T KNOW WHAT YOU'RE LOOKING FOR.

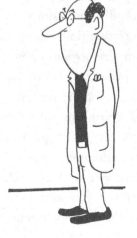

What are the ethical limitations of clinical trials?

Few clinical trials have the evaluation of safety as their prime objective. Such trials would raise ethical issues. If an important safety problem is suspected, it would be difficult to design a clinical trial without violating the fundamental principles of the Declaration of Helsinki.[9]

Pregnant women are often excluded from participating in clinical trials of new drugs. Including them is considered an unnecessary risk to the fetus. Clearly, it would be entirely unethical to enroll women during the first trimester specifically to determine potential teratogenic effects of a new drug. Possible exceptions are clinical trials designed to evaluate interventions that are likely to benefit mother and/or infant. One such example includes trials that assessed the value of various regimens in preventing vertical transmission of HIV infection from mother to child.

The exclusion of pregnant women from clinical trials of new drugs creates an information vacuum. Many drugs are approved and marketed without any prior information on teratogenic effects in humans. Animal toxicity studies are not always good surrogates. Mechanisms are in place, however, to gather this information after drug approval from non-experimental studies. A few countries, including Sweden, have a comprehensive, well-functioning registry with confidential data on mothers' exposure to drugs and on diagnosed birth defects. A recent publication from the Swedish registry reported an almost doubling in risk of cardiovascular birth defects among mothers using erythromycin early during pregnancy.[4] This antibiotic has been on the market for more than half a century.

Another ethical issue relates to the use of established standard drugs in patient populations enrolled in a clinical trial. Withholding such therapy from study subjects would be a violation of the Declaration of Helsinki. It is very unlikely that an IRB would approve a clinical trial in patients with heart failure unless all study subjects were given an ACE inhibitor, or angiotensin receptor blocker (ARB), the rationale being that a proven beneficial intervention should never be withheld. In this instance, any new heart failure medication must be evaluated in conjunction with standard treatment, despite the fact that ACE inhibitors and ARBs are substantially underprescribed for the treatment of heart failure.[2] The reason for this is that whereas the conduct of clinical trials is regulated, the practice of medicine is not.

Key Points

- ⚬ Safety assessment represents a potential weakness of randomized clinical trials.
- ⚬ Adverse effects with a true incidence of less than one in 1,000 are rarely detected.
- ⚬ Due to short trial durations, adverse effects appearing a year or more after treatment initiation often go undetected.
- ⚬ Unexpected adverse effects, even if common, are seldom detected.
- ⚬ Ethical considerations based on the Declaration of Helsinki may limit the scientific questions that clinical trials can address.

"If the world were perfect, it wouldn't be"
(Y. Berra)

Chapter 5

Do meta-analyses provide the ultimate truth?

Well-written and well-balanced review articles represent important sources of information for busy professionals, who find it demanding to keep up with the increasing flow of scientific information in a growing number of specialty journals. Even scientists with expertise in specific therapeutic areas find it difficult to stay up-to-date. One of the major challenges in perusing the clinical trials literature concerns how to integrate multiple clinical trial results, some of which appear to be, at least in part, contradictory.

Although most overviews provide an objective and condensed picture of a complex topic, biases that plague individual clinical trials can also affect systematic clinical trial reviews. The author(s) may selectively highlight or down-play individual studies. Bias can enter the picture as soon as there is an element of judgment. Fortunately, facts have a refreshing way of limiting the scope of speculation. It is always a good idea for the reader to determine if the authors of review articles are independent scientists as discussed in Chapter 20. Loyalty does not invalidate a review, but readers should be alerted to the possibility of a partisan slant, especially concerning controversial issues for which the data are not clear. Authors may also have reasons to defend long-held positions.

Meta-analysis, a special type of review article, emerged in the medical literature during the 1980s and has since gained enormous recognition and popularity. Also known as an overview or a "pooled" analysis, meta-analysis is a database-oriented publication that uses formal statistical methods to combine outcome results from multiple studies of related interventions.

What are the advantages with meta-analyses?
Meta-analyses have several important advantages. Combining trial results increases the number of patients for the analysis and, in turn, increases the statistical power for evaluating treatment effects. Thus, more moderate treatment differences, which may be clinically important, stand a greater chance of being

detected and declared statistically significant. Pooled analysis can also identify subgroups of patients who may respond favorably (or unfavorably) to a given therapy. Combining related trials from different geographic regions, or from different countries, enriches the variability of patient groups, thereby providing a more robust test of how far the intervention results can be generalized. In addition, meta-analyses tend to neutralize the extreme findings (positive or negative) from individual trials.

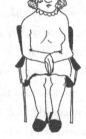 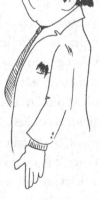

— MRS. LAWLESS, THIS DRUG WORKED IN A META-ANALYSIS OF 90,000 PATIENTS.
— DOES THAT MEAN IT WILL WORK FOR ME?

What are the disadvantages?

There are some drawbacks to the meta-analytic approach. One strength also represents a source of weakness. Combining *all* trial results, published and unpublished, leads to the pooling of data from both methodologically sound and perhaps poorly conducted trials. *Publication bias* represents another potential problem.[6] Articles with neutral or unfavorable findings may never be published, sometimes due to investigator "inertia," but probably more often due to the lackluster results. In addition, trial reports without statistically significant positive results have a hard time finding their way into leading medical journals. The under-representation of neutral or negative trial results in a meta-analysis or any other systematic review tends to overestimate the beneficial effects of a therapy.

A recent report noted that of the 13 trials of selective serotonin reuptake inhibitors (SSRIs) that have been conducted in adolescents,[9] three reported favorable results for the SSRIs while 10 showed no difference compared to placebo. The former were published in high profile journals, the latter remained unpublished.

Concerns about inclusion of data in a meta-analysis from clinical trials of varying quality have led to the use of quality grading criteria, which define trial standards. This system permits limiting the inclusion of only trials meeting specific standards in the meta-analysis. Inclusion may also be restricted to certain patient groups, conditions, types of interventions, classes of drugs, treatment duration, etc. While these restrictions may be rational, exclusion of trials, for any reason, might itself introduce bias. Though the meta-analyst is aware of the trial results, it is important that the entry criteria are not dependent on the trial results. In fact, we should not forget that all meta-analyses are in that sense *post hoc*. The postmaster who managed to place his postal bets on the horses that had already won the races was convicted, as discussed in Chapter 8.

A comprehensive meta-analysis goes well beyond tabulating published results. Many published trials may not include certain outcomes of interest to the meta-analyst, or certain outcomes may not have been measured and recorded in a particular trial. Only inquiries directed to the trial authors can clarify whether the data pertinent to the meta-analysis exist and, if they do, whether the respective trial investigator(s) will release these data to the meta-analyst. Such requests for additional information are time-consuming and are not always well received. Another reason for inquiry is to obtain outcome data from randomized patients who were excluded from the final trial report.

Although often not readily apparent, similar trials may have important differences: disease severity among enrolled patients, concomitant treatment, different drugs from the same class, drug dosing, methods and time points for assessing treatment effects, and compliance. Critics of meta-analysis question the value of combining *all* individual trials into a "composite" trial. They claim that the technique combines apples, oranges, bananas and, occasionally, lemons into a single product, the quality of which is difficult to assess.

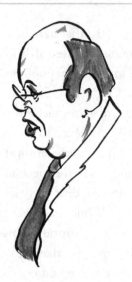

— THE ACCURATE TIME IS
NOT NECESSARILY THE
AVERAGE OF SEVERAL
INACCURATE WATCHES.

How do findings from meta-analyses compare with those from subsequent large trials?

One criticism of meta-analyses is that they often include a large number of fairly small clinical trials conducted for a variety of reasons. Because smaller trials are less likely to be published compared to larger trials, many of these studies may be overlooked. However, even findings from meta-analyses of large trials can be misleading. This notion is supported by the findings of a study that compared the results of meta-analyses to those of subsequent large trials (sample size of at least 1,000 patients).[5] Among 19 meta-analyses, the authors found 12 subsequently published large trials focusing on the same scientific question. In two-thirds of these, the findings were inconsistent with the meta-analyses.

Two cases illustrate that reported results from meta-analyses of a large number of small trials and results from large clinical trials may differ. First, although intravenous corticosteroids have been used to treat head injuries for three decades, scientific documentation supporting this therapy is sparse. A meta-analysis of the available trial evidence reported in 1997 included 13 trials and about 2,000 patients.[1] The point estimate for the relative reduction in mortality was 9% but the 95% confidence interval was wide, ranging from - 26 to +12%. This lack of good sound evidence was the impetus for a large, definitive international trial. The design of this placebo-controlled trial, CRASH,[3] called for a total sample size of 20,000, which was estimated to provide adequate statistical power to detect a 2% absolute survival difference. The independent data monitoring and ethics committee recommended that the trial be terminated when results were available on about 10,000 patients. Surprisingly, the two-week mortality was higher in the corticosteroid group (21.1% vs. 17.9%; 18% relative difference). The accompanying commentary projected that corticosteroid treatment may have caused approximately 5,000 unnecessary deaths annually.[8]

Second, in critically ill patients, an inverse relationship exists between serum albumin concentration and mortality. Administration of albumin solutions is commonplace in intensive care units. A systematic review of 30 randomized clinical trials that included approximately 1,400 patients was published in 1998.[2] The relative risk of mortality in the albumin-treated group was 88% higher than among the controls. The absolute difference in mortality was 6%, which indicated that for every 17 albumin-treated patients, there was one excess death. This observation generated worldwide attention, but did not discourage investigators in Australia and New Zealand from embarking on a placebo-controlled trial of albumin in 7,000 patients.[7] At the conclusion of the trial, there was no mortality difference between the treatment groups.

These two cases demonstrate that meta-analyses, which incorporate considerable numbers of smaller trials, may overestimate benefits or risks of commonly used treatments.

What is a cumulative meta-analysis?

The cumulative meta-analysis is a special form of meta-analysis with similar strengths and weaknesses. After a meta-analysis of the first two trials, the analysis is repeated adding one trial at a time in the order of their date of publication. This approach addresses the question "When did we know?" Experience has shown that convincing scientific evidence is typically available long before the medical profession recognizes it and responds by modifying treatment guidelines. A similar delay to acceptance also applies to adverse effects. A recent cumulative meta-analysis[4] concluded that the increased risk of heart attacks attributed to rofecoxib (Vioxx) was, or should have been, known years before the drug was withdrawn from the market.

Key Points

- ⚬⤙ Meta-analyses increase the statistical power to detect moderate treatment differences.
- ⚬⤙ They may allow detection of patient subgroups that respond differently to an intervention.
- ⚬⤙ Publication bias leads to under-representation of neutral or negative trials, resulting in overestimation of benefits.
- ⚬⤙ Consistency between findings from meta-analyses and large trials is not perfect.
- ⚬⤙ The cumulative meta-analysis tells us when the answer "is in."

*"The chain is only as strong
as its weakest link"*

Chapter 6

What are the strengths of observational studies?

Observational studies can provide valuable information about treatment effects, especially with regard to adverse drug reactions. Compared to clinical trials, observational studies have two major advantages — greater access to large, diverse, groups of patients, and relatively quick data collection and analysis. They are an important alternative when it is not feasible to conduct a randomized trial or when it is believed to be unethical to do so, as discussed in Chapter 4. Observational studies allow us to compare outcomes in users and non-users of a particular drug.

What are the types of observational studies?
There are seven main types:
1. Case reports are individual patient cases. They are the simplest form of an observational study.
2. Case series are compilations of several case reports.
3. Cross-sectional studies are based on measurements obtained at a single time point with no follow-up.
4. Case-control studies compare subjects who have a particular condition (cases) to those without that condition (controls). Investigators seek to determine after the fact (i.e., retrospectively) whether differences in past exposure to one or more drugs could explain why cases suffered the condition and controls did not.
5. Cohort studies follow groups of individuals forward in time (i.e., prospectively), and compare the risk of disease or disease complications among users and non-users of a drug.
6. Registry studies typically make use of the electronic medical records of patients from large healthcare providers.
7. Qualitative studies, which may be interview- or questionnaire-based, focus on evaluating patients' reactions to an illness and its treatment.

Are case reports of any value?

In 1983, Venning[5] investigated how major adverse effects of prescription drugs were first noticed. Surprisingly, of 18 well recognized serious adverse drug reactions referenced, 13 were first published as case reports.

A classic example was published in 1961 as a Letter to the Editor by an obstetrician in Sydney.[4] Over a six-week period, he noted that three newborn infants had the same rare limb defect. He suspected that there was a link between the mothers' use of thalidomide and the congenital abnormality. Unfortunately, more than 10,000 affected children were born worldwide before this association was confirmed and the drug removed from the market.

Other case reports have led to a faster regulatory response and drug withdrawal, e.g, the association between Guillain-Barré syndrome and the antidepressant zimeldine (Zelmid) and the connection between serious ventricular arrhythmias and the antihistamine terfenadine (Seldane). Although the clinical value of case reports is usually limited, they can sometimes give important warning signals for serious, unexpected or rare adverse events.

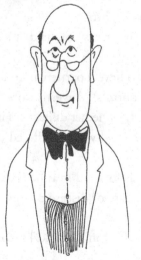

— I HAVE THE DISTINCT IMPRESSION THAT RARE ADVERSE REACTIONS ARE BECOMING MORE AND MORE COMMON.

Occasionally, case reports bring attention to rare favorable drug actions. In studies of the beta-blocker propranolol (Inderal), some patients reported a reduction in migraine episodes while others noted decreased tremors. These case reports led to controlled studies and two new indications for propranolol (Inderal). Similarly, some angina pectoris patients involved in a trial of sildenafil (Viagra) reported a favorable effect on erectile dysfunction.

What are the strengths of case series?
The likelihood of false or random associations that may be drawn from individual case reports diminishes with an increasing number of confirmatory observations in a case series. Sometimes a case series may be generated prospectively, with investigators waiting for additional cases to appear in their practice or in the medical literature before reporting their observations.

Other case series document the effects of an intervention, often surgical, in an uncontrolled series of patients (i.e., no comparison group). The findings, if favorable, can provide a strong rationale for conducting a controlled clinical trial. This is the "proof of concept" approach that is often taken by the pharmaceutical industry during early drug development.

How useful are cross-sectional studies for evaluation of treatment effects?
Cross-sectional studies have several advantages. First, a large number of measurements can be taken quickly and at a modest cost. Second, since the researchers are collecting the data, they have control over study methodology as well as patient selection.

The cross-sectional study provides a good first step towards exploring possible associations. A comparison of long-term users of a given drug with carefully matched non-users can provide important preliminary information that could lead to further confirmatory studies.

What are the advantages of case-control studies?
Case-control studies are retrospective. The cases are usually patients who, over a period of time, have been diagnosed with a specific condition or complication. The controls are recruited from the same population and should be as similar

as possible to the cases, with the exception that they do not have the condition being evaluated. Information on prior drug exposures in the two study groups is collected and compared. Case-control studies are particularly useful for evaluating uncommon conditions or unusual drug reactions. They can be completed inexpensively and within a reasonable timeframe. The association between drug exposure and a specific condition is expressed as an "*Odds Ratio*" (OR), which, for uncommon events, is a good approximation of the "*Relative Risk*" (RR).

In a case-control study of women aged 18 to 49 years,[3] it was reported that the use of phenylpropanolamine for weight reduction was associated with an odds ratio of 16.6 (95% confidence interval (CI)1.5-182; p = 0.02) for subarachnoid or intracerebral hemorrhage; for the indication common cold, the OR was 3.1 (95% CI 0.86-11.5; p = 0.08). If these study findings are true, is the temporary symptomatic relief of a common cold worth the risk of a rare but potentially fatal adverse event?

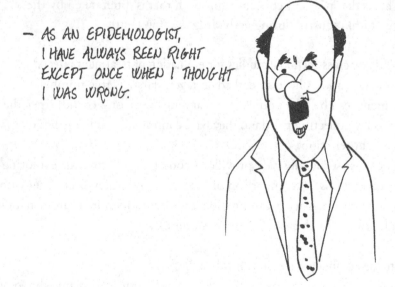

— AS AN EPIDEMIOLOGIST, I HAVE ALWAYS BEEN RIGHT EXCEPT ONCE WHEN I THOUGHT I WAS WRONG.

What are the strengths of cohort studies?

The main advantage of cohort studies is that they are conducted prospectively. Consequently, the researchers can determine the precise population to be studied, the methods of collecting the data, and data quality. If patient follow-up is intensive and prolonged, these studies can be more costly than other observational studies. A classic cohort study was initiated among British doctors more than half a century ago.[1] Approximately 35,000 male physicians responded to a survey of their smoking habits. In a series of articles over five decades, these investigators observed a marked increase in mortality among those who smoked.[2] Habitual smoking shortened the lifespan by about 10 years.

What is the potential value of disease registries?

We have recently seen an increase in the number of large disease- and condition-specific registries, as well as registries of patients undergoing particular procedures. These are often part of larger electronic databases, which link to pharmacy records. These have been helpful in identifying both favorable and unfavorable long-term effects of various interventions. For example, information on drug utilization by pregnant women has proven valuable when linked to a registry of congenital birth defects. Registries may also rule out suspected associations.

What is the role of qualitative studies?

Randomized clinical trials and observational studies rarely consider individual patients' perceptions or preferences. Qualitative studies fill this void. One must not forget that patients may regard risks and benefits very differently, and patients with the same medical condition may have very different symptoms, as well as completely different thresholds of tolerance for these symptoms. Some patients with asthma may suffer primarily from exertion dyspnea, while others have difficulty coping with dry cough or insomnia due to nocturnal attacks. Any trial evaluating asthma interventions for symptomatic relief ought to focus especially on what is most important to individual patients. Patient perspectives and expectations should be taken into account when designing trials to evaluate interventions.

Key Points

- ⚷ Compared to clinical trials, observational studies offer greater access to large, diverse populations, provide a quicker result, and cost less.
- ⚷ They serve as an alternative when randomized trials are not possible or are unethical.
- ⚷ They are important for detecting adverse reactions that are uncommon, unexpected or occur late.
- ⚷ They may be descriptive in nature or they may compare drug users to non-users.
- ⚷ They are valuable for generating new hypotheses.

"You can observe a lot by watching"

(Y. Berra)

Chapter 7

What are the weaknesses of observational studies?

There are also inherent weaknesses with observational studies when they are used to evaluate treatment effects. Potential problems relate to various biases, the quality of the data, and the often exploratory nature of the analysis.

Potential biases

Retrospective studies that rely on participant recollection of events, behaviors, etc. are susceptible to *recall bias*, since cases may have a biased recollection of drug exposure than controls.

Group comparability, a key element of the randomized clinical trial, is a concern in observational studies. If the use of one treatment or another in patients with a given condition occurred randomly, then comparing users and non-users would be valid. However, users often receive a particular intervention based on the severity of symptoms or the risk of disease complications. Patients with a milder form of disease may take less potent drugs, or may receive no treatment at all. This so-called "*indication bias*" must be considered in observational studies.

Conversely, drug use can also be a marker of "healthy" users — patients who are less sick. For decades, we were led to believe that hormone replacement therapy (HRT) reduced the risk of coronary events. This information came from observational studies, which showed a lower coronary risk among users compared to non-users of HRT.[3] Although reports indicated that users were healthier, had fewer risk factors and saw their physicians more often, the observation was not accepted until randomized clinical trials[1,7] provided no evidence that HRT is cardioprotective. This type of *selection bias* may also account for the observation that users of lipid-lowering statins run a lower risk of developing Alzheimer's disease (AD) than non-users.[2,4,6] AD is less common in subjects with higher education and/or higher socioeconomic status, and this segment of the population is more likely to be prescribed and remain adherent to preventive measures, to have health insurance, and/or be able to pay for expensive treatments. Moreover, cognitively impaired subjects may not be prescribed preventive medications. Only well-designed clinical trials can resolve this debate.

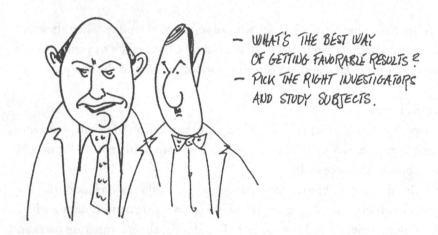

What are the specific limitations of observational studies?

Although case reports and case series may provide an early warning of drug toxicity, they also can cause "false alarms." Unexpected or serious adverse events that occur during a particular treatment are not necessarily related to that treatment. However, an analysis of 47 early case reports did conclude that the majority of suspected adverse events were subsequently confirmed.[5] A prudent approach is to wait and see if similar additional cases are reported. It has been suggested that publication of a suspected treatment-induced adverse event should be delayed until at least three cases have occurred.

The principal limitation of cross-sectional studies is their inability to address temporal and causal relationships. If users of a drug have a medical condition, it may not be possible to distinguish whether they were prescribed the drug because of their condition, or whether their condition was drug-induced.

Case-control studies are also susceptible to the same biases. Lack of comparability between the groups being evaluated remains a key concern.

Stratified analyses (for example, by severity of illness) may reduce the impact of indication bias.

Unlike retrospective studies, prospective cohort studies should not involve a recall bias. Although they are still subject to both indication and selection biases, prospective cohort studies can be valuable in exploring favorable and unfavorable treatment effects.

Qualitative studies are open-ended and descriptive in nature. They yield preliminary, but subjective, information about risk tolerance and treatment preferences.

Key Points

- The retrospective nature of observational studies may limit their data quality.
- Cases may recall drug exposure differently than controls (*recall bias*).
- Users are often different from non-users (*indication bias*).
- Group comparability is a critical factor in observational studies (*selection bias*).

"Even the sun has its spots"

Chapter 8

Were the scientific questions stated in advance?

An exploratory study examines the available data and generates a new hypothesis that needs to be tested. A clinical trial determines prospectively whether this hypothesis is true and provides an estimate of the treatment effect. It is essential that in a clinical trial, the number of hypotheses are limited and stated in advance. The following quotation illustrates the distinction:[4]

> "Once there was a punter (gambler) who backed more winners than would have been expected by chance (p < 0.00001). He was brought to trial and convicted because he had misused his position as village postmaster to antedate his postal bets after he knew which horses had won their races. The jury felt it was wrong for an individual who knew the results to pretend to play a game of chance with the bookmakers."

An exploratory study would describe the various races and the characteristics of the horses by the order they reached the finish line. This information could then be used to generate ideas about which horses represented good bets in future races. A randomized clinical trial is like a horse race that tests the generated hypothesis. Hypotheses (bets) must be "placed" prior to performing the trial (running the race).

Why is *a priori* testing important?

The principle of *a priori* hypothesis testing is critical because testing for statistical significance remains valid only if hypotheses are stated in advance. Occasionally, investigators believe they should have the same advantage that the postmaster had, namely allowing the outcome of the trial to determine on which hypotheses to bet. Like the postmaster, these investigators should be censured since they ignore basic scientific and statistical principles.

Good science requires that a clinical trial has one pre-specified, *primary* hypothesis. Additional *secondary* hypotheses are permissible, but these usually relate to the primary question as "variations of the primary theme." Regulatory authorities routinely require that a clearly defined primary hypothesis is stated in the protocol before a trial starts. Unfortunately, regulatory agencies in some other countries are less demanding.

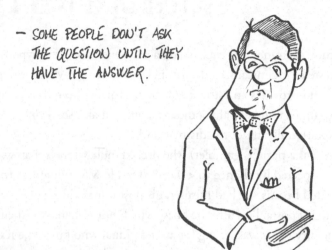

There are several ways to "cheat" the bookmakers: stating a vague or ill-defined hypothesis that remains unspecified until after the race; stating many hypotheses, so-called "multiple hypothesis testing," which is similar to placing bets on every horse in the race; and ignoring the *a priori* rule of specifying the hypothesis before the trial and hoping that no one will notice.

In a New Zealand study evaluating asthma treatment,[6] regular and "as needed" administration of fenoterol were compared using a non-standardized combination of respiratory flow, symptomatic improvement and drug use. The investigators reported that a significantly greater number of patients deteriorated over 24 weeks when given regular inhaled beta-agonist treatment compared to on-demand treatment. Unfortunately, the "home-made" criteria for assessing drug effectiveness had not been specified in advance. Often it is impossible for readers to know when investigators play the "postmaster's game," even if the study is reported in a highly reputable journal. Without access to the trial protocol or a design paper, one cannot know for certain whether the investigators clearly stated a limited number of *a priori* hypotheses or whether the hypotheses were subsequently defined, or possibly redefined, to fit the results. In a survey comparing trial protocols to journal publications, major discrepancies were observed among nineteen of 48 (40%) trials, in terms of which primary outcomes were pre-specified.[2]

Another survey of 102 Danish trials observed incomplete reporting of outcomes reflecting efficacy and safety in 50% and 65% of the trials, respectively.[1] At least one primary outcome was introduced, changed, or omitted in 62% of the trials.

The issue of multiple hypothesis testing can be illustrated with another analogy. Anyone playing a single number on a fair fortune wheel with 20 numbers knows that his/her chance of winning is, on average, one in twenty or 5%. This chance increases with the number of bets. Clinical trial investigators also know that the odds of winning increase if they place several bets, or if they define multiple hypotheses. Another way of increasing the chance of winning is to spin the wheel several times — for instance, to evaluate subjects at each of multiple follow-up visits during a trial. Normally, one places new bets with every spin. Some investigators, however, expect free spins. If the study protocol has five pre-specified hypotheses and subjects return for four evaluation visits, the number of statistical tests is twenty. Even if the treatment has no beneficial effect, the chance of declaring a positive effect is 5% per test (p=0.05). Thus, the probability is very high that at least one bet will turn out to be a "winning" statistically significant number. The issue of multiple hypothesis testing is discussed further in Chapter 22.

— A BRILLIANT ANSWER,
 BUT WHAT WAS THE QUESTION?

We cannot allow the practice of medicine to be influenced by chance findings or *post hoc* "interpretations" of the results. Clinicians must rely on their clinical experience as well as their common sense to uncover violations of the principles of hypothesis testing. Red flags may include the use of unusual or illogical composites, e.g., outcome measures that have uncertain clinical relevance. Preferred outcomes are those that both clinicians and patients consider important.

Is clinical trial registration the solution?

In the past, readers of a clinical trial report rarely had access to trial protocols. This made it difficult to uncover any modifications of the pre-specified hypotheses. The situation changed in 2000 with the establishment of a U.S. web-based registry, "ClinicalTrials.gov."[8] A new law now mandates registration of effectiveness trials for "serious or life-threatening" conditions that will involve submission of investigational new drug applications to the FDA. Since May of 2004, a similar requirement has been in effect in Europe.[5] An important difference between these registries is that the U.S. one is open to the public, while the European registry remains closed. Since September of 2005, leading medical journals[3] have mandated protocol registration if they are to publish the trial results. The World Health Organization is in the process of setting up an International Clinical Trials Registry Platform that will involve a minimum trial registration dataset of 20 items.[7]

Compliance with the U.S. regulations is high for non-profit organizations, but varies among pharmaceutical companies.[8] High proportions of meaningless entries in the "Intervention Name" field, 21 and 11%, respectively, were noted for two major companies. The "Primary Outcome" field was only completed 3% of the time by a third company.

Key Points

- A clinical trial should have *one* pre-specified, primary hypothesis.
- When the results for the primary hypothesis are not significant, be cautious if the focus is shifted to a secondary endpoint, or one that is defined *post hoc*.
- Without access to the trial protocol, readers of medical journals have no way of knowing what the pre-specified primary and secondary hypotheses were.
- As of July, 2005, leading medical journals only publish articles from pre-registered clinical trials.

"You've got to be careful if you don't know where you're going 'cause you might not get there"

(Y. Berra)

Chapter 9

Were the treatment groups comparable initially?

The purpose of a controlled clinical trial is to compare two or more treatment approaches. It is important that the treatment groups are comparable at the beginning of the study and that any group differences are identified. Randomization is and should be the preferred standard process by which patients are allocated to treatment groups. It assures that each patient has the same chance of being assigned to either the intervention or the control group. Randomization not only guarantees the validity of the statistical tests but also maximizes study group comparability with regard to known and unknown prognostic factors at baseline. The process also removes investigator bias in the treatment allocation of patients.

What is randomization?
Randomization, by definition, randomly assigns patients to the treatment groups. Often compared to a coin toss, the actual randomization process is usually accomplished by use of random number tables or computer programs. It is important that neither the investigator nor the patient knows the random assignment prior to the patient's decision whether or not to enroll. In the older clinical trials literature, one can find examples of trials that allocated participants to treatment groups according to the date of enrollment. Participants enrolled on odd dates received treatment A; patients enrolled on even dates were allocated to treatment B. This is not a form of randomization, since the physician knew the treatment assignment and could control who got enrolled. Even subconsciously, an investigator favoring treatment A could selectively enroll sicker patients into group B and allow lower-risk patients to enter group A. Comparisons of baseline characteristics in trials using this form of "randomization" have confirmed the existence of major investigator biases. Investigators who may have

opinions about the therapy under study are poor substitutes for random tables and computer programs.

Does randomization guarantee group comparability?

On average, randomization produces comparable groups. In individual trials, especially small ones, even the most effective randomization scheme cannot guarantee group comparability. Although it is not reassuring to have group imbalances, they do not invalidate the trial or its results. One way of minimizing imbalances among study groups, especially with regard to important or critical baseline characteristics that are believed to correlate with treatment response or outcome, is through *stratified randomization*. In this technique each characteristic has its own separate randomization scheme. Common stratification factors are age, disease severity, and clinic (in multicenter trials). In cardiovascular studies, one may want to ensure a similar distribution of patients with diabetes

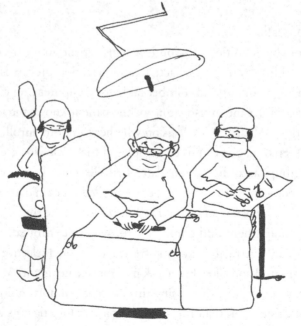

and heart failure, or in studies of gastric ulcer one may want to stratify on smoking status and ulcer diameter.

Simple randomization in small trials of 150-200 patients or less may result in substantial group imbalances by chance alone. Such imbalances, which can favor either group, may contribute to observed treatment-control group differences. For this reason, the FDA often requires that findings from one trial be confirmed in a second independent trial of similar design, unless the treatment differences are very large.

Can group differences be controlled for?

Another way of dealing with group imbalance at baseline is by statistical adjustment for the imbalance of prognostic factors across treatment groups at the end of the trial. These adjustments are based on certain assumptions, which may or may not be valid. Since a number of prognostic factors may remain unknown or unmeasured, there is no assurance that all critical factors are included in the adjustment. Some skepticism of this procedure seems appropriate, especially if the unadjusted and adjusted analyses lead to different conclusions, but this rarely occurs. The most conservative approach is to accept the finding that shows the least difference between the treatment and control groups. Statistical adjustment works well, so long as prognostic factors are known and are reliably and accurately measured. This is not always the case.

What should the reader look for?

The distribution of baseline prognostic factors among the study groups should be included in one of the early tables of a trial report. It is important for the reader to review this table to obtain a sense of group comparability. Group differences are very unusual in large trials. Therefore, it came as no surprise when the reported differences in both mean baseline systolic and diastolic blood pressures in the "Captopril Prevention Project"[1] attracted a lot of attention.[2] In this trial of about 11,000 hypertensive subjects, the 2-3 mm Hg difference suggested tampering with the randomization process. The probability that these differences were due to chance alone was less than one in a million.

Many prognostic factors that influence the outcome of a trial may be unknown or may have not been measured. Chance itself sometimes favors the intervention and sometimes the control group. Imbalances of this kind may help explain why two similar trials sometimes yield different results.

Key Points

o━ Treatment group comparability at baseline is an essential feature of clinical trials.

o━ Randomization is the preferred process by which patients are allocated to treatment groups, since, on average, it produces comparable groups.

o━ Simple randomization may result in substantial group imbalances in smaller trials (150-200 patients or less).

o━ Stratified randomization is one way of minimizing imbalances for important patient characteristics.

o━ Statistical adjustment for baseline imbalances of prognostic factors is another way of dealing with group imbalances.

o━ Since group imbalances may exist even if the known prognostic factors are evenly distributed, exercise caution in accepting medical breakthroughs based on a single trial.

"A good beginning makes a good ending"

Chapter 10

Why is blinding/masking so important?

Investigator or patient knowledge of treatment assignment almost inevitably leads to biased assessment. One way to minimize this is to keep the investigator and the study subjects blinded, or masked, to the identity of the treatment assignment. In a *single-blind* trial, only the patients are unaware of which intervention they receive. In a *double-blind* trial, the investigator and associated trial personnel, as well as the patients, are blinded to treatment identity. A double-blind design is preferred for most outcomes. The more subjective the endpoint, the more important blinding becomes. However, many types of trials — for example surgical procedures or dietary modification — do not lend themselves to blinding. In trials where blinding is not feasible, the risk of biased assessment can threaten the integrity of the study, necessitating the use of special bias-reducing techniques.

Most outcomes, beneficial or harmful, have some element of subjectivity. Knowledge of treatment group assignment may influence the investigator's evaluation and classification of the treatment response. Additionally, the investigator may prescribe compensatory or concomitant treatments that could diminish any treatment difference between the intervention and the control groups.

Study subjects aware of their treatment allocation may also have preconceived notions or expectations when they enter a research project. Many are also anxious to please their physician or to give the "right" answer.

In general, clinical trials of pharmacologic agents should employ a double-blind design. Special efforts should be made to ensure a good physical match between the active drug and its corresponding placebo or control agent. Differences in taste, odor or color can cause unblinding. Although pharmacologic effects such as changes in heart rate or blood pressure or side effects such as tremor, constipation or dry mouth may reveal the identity of the blinded medications in a subset of patients, this does not justify abandoning the double-blind trial design.

In trials evaluating surgical, behavioral, or physiotherapy interventions where blinding is impractical, efforts should be made to rely on a third party for independent and blinded assessment of intervention effects. The use of a third party may also be important in trials of drugs that are very difficult to mask. The Heart and Estrogen/progestin Replacement Study[1] relied on gynecological staff to assess breast discomfort and vaginal bleeding and separate clinical center staff for determining cardiovascular outcomes.

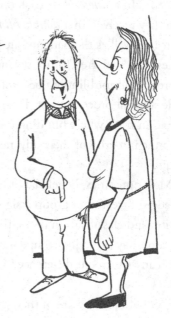

Why is blinding so important?

In the 1970s, a group of investigators from the National Institutes of Health conducted a double-blind, placebo-controlled, 9-month trial that evaluated the prophylactic and therapeutic effects of vitamin C (ascorbic acid) for the common cold.[2] Three hundred NIH employees were enrolled. While the number of episodes of the common cold was similar in both groups at the conclusion of the study, the intervention group reported shorter duration of colds. Investigation showed that a proportion of the enrollees could not resist the temptation to break the blind by tasting or even identifying the content of their capsules. When the investigators analyzed the data by subjects who remained unaware of their treatment assignment, no difference existed in the duration of colds. Among those enrollees who had broken the blind, the duration was shorter in subjects who knew they were taking vitamin C and longer in subjects who knew they were on placebo. This example suggests that expectations about the treatment may influence the subject's perception or reporting of treatment effects (in this case, duration of the cold). It also illustrates that people who are curious by nature (for example, scientists), may not be the best study subjects for a double-blind trial!

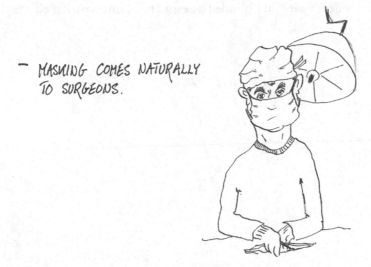

What are the disadvantages of open design?

Knowledge of treatment assignment can consciously or subconsciously influence decisions about terminating study medication, prescribing concomitant interventions, classifying study events, and reporting adverse effects. If these actions differ between study groups, bias is introduced. The so-called PROBE (Prospective, Randomized, Open, Blinded Endpoint) design does not address most of these biases. However, the reliance on an independent committee of experts blinded to group assignment for classification of study events is a positive feature.

Key Points

o⟍ Most outcomes, beneficial or harmful, have some element of subjectivity.

o⟍ Keeping study subjects and study investigators blinded to the identity of the treatment assignment lowers the risk of biased reporting and assessment.

o⟍ Investigators aware of treatment assignment may differentially prescribe concomitant treatments.

o⟍ Study subjects aware of their treatment allocation may wish to please their physician by giving the "right" answer.

o⟍ If blinding is impractical, a third party ("a blinded observer") may be used for independent and blinded assessment of intervention effects.

"In the dark, all shades are gray"

Chapter 11

How is symptomatic improvement measured?

Only patients can accurately assess how they really feel. One should question the findings of any clinical trial that depends on a physician's assessment of the severity of a patient's symptoms such as itching, heartburn or insomnia.

Unfortunately, many investigators and sponsors are reluctant to accept patient self-reports as primary outcomes. However, when the objective of treatment is to alleviate symptoms or to improve well-being, a subjective but relevant measure has more meaning than one which is objective but irrelevant. Findings from clinical trials using patient self-reports are usually valid, provided that treatment assignment was effectively blinded.

The unwillingness to use patient-reported symptoms as major trial outcomes comes, in part, from the difficulty in measuring the severity of the symptoms and their improvement. Symptoms can be hard to define, let alone quantify Symptoms are perceived differently by different patients, and many symptoms come and go. If a single disease results in multiple symptoms, which one, or ones, should be evaluated to determine the efficacy of an intervention?

Which symptoms are most relevant?

It is important to limit the number of questions patients are asked and to focus on those symptoms they perceive as the most troublesome or that are the most responsive to the therapy. Epigastric pain is the most frequently reported symptom for patients with an acute duodenal ulcer. Most patients want rapid pain relief and actual healing of the ulcer is a secondary concern. Therefore, it makes sense that patients' self-reported perception of epigastric pain should be the primary outcome in studies evaluating an acute treatment for duodenal ulcers. However, trials of maintenance therapy for duodenal ulcer should evaluate not only long-term symptomatic relief, but also the extent of ulcer healing and the reduced risk of recurrence and complications, such as bleeding or perforation.

A similar situation exists for trials of anti-asthmatic treatments. In an

asthma attack, exertional dyspnea and nocturnal orthopnea are the most
troublesome symptoms for the patient; clinical trials of acute treatment should
focus on those symptoms. In contrast, trials evaluating the effectiveness of long-
term maintenance therapy need to assess the prevention of acute exacerbations
and disease progression, so it is appropriate to measure complication rates,
changes in pulmonary function and, in more advanced disease stages, survival.

The reliance on functional measures to evaluate disease severity can be
misleading. In patients with benign prostatic hyperplasia, urodynamic studies
help to quantify the degree of urinary obstruction, which causes a weak stream
and hesitancy; but this correlates poorly with the severity of urgency and
nocturia, which are the more troublesome symptoms for the patient. Thus,
urodynamic measures have limited value in assessing the symptomatic actions of
an intervention.

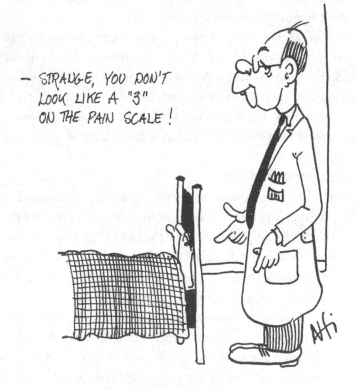

How is symptom severity measured?

Symptom severity can be measured in a number of ways. One approach is to ask the patient to rate the symptom(s) according to a scale defined with numbers and corresponding descriptions, such as 0 = none, 1 = mild, 2 = moderate or 3 = severe. Alternatively, the patient can indicate his/her perception of *change* in symptom severity from an earlier time point, usually prior to starting the treatment being evaluated; for example, marked improvement, moderate or slight improvement, no change, slight or moderate worsening, or marked worsening. Although these scales provide a means of communicating the results of a study, the precise interpretation will depend on the previous experiences of the reader. Severe, moderate, or mild improvement may engender different expectations in different people.

If there are too few steps on a severity scale, clinically important changes in symptoms may be missed, whereas if there are too many, the patient may have problems differentiating between subtle differences in verbal descriptions. The optimal number of steps appears to be five or seven.

Another method of quantifying symptoms employs a visual analog scale (VAS), which usually comprises a 100 mm line with verbal descriptions attached to either end; for instance, 'no pain' and 'intolerable pain' at opposing ends of the line. There are no verbal cues between the two poles. Patients are asked to mark the line at the point that they believe reflects their symptom severity. A numerical score (the number of millimeters from one end of the scale) can then be assigned to represent the symptom severity. This continuous scale, which shows all values between 0 and 100 mm, is easy to complete and is unaffected by a patient's interpretation of verbal descriptions. It is also more sensitive, as a statistically significant difference in this continuous measure can often be demonstrated in fewer patients. The major disadvantage of the VAS is interpreting and communicating the clinical relevance of a scale change. What exactly does it mean if a new analgesic reduces pain, on average, from 58 to 43 mm? Also, 5 millimeters in the middle of the scale does not necessarily represent the same change in symptom severity as 5 millimeters near the poles.

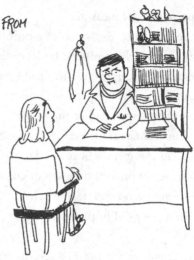

Key Points

- Subjective symptoms are best assessed by patients themselves.
- Patients with the same diagnosis may suffer from different symptoms.
- What may be of little concern to one patient is troublesome to another.
- Changes in VAS scores lend themselves to statistical analysis more easily, but their clinical importance is uncertain.
- Rating scales are more patient-important but have analytic limitations.

"The customer is always right"

Chapter 12

Is it really possible to assess quality of life?

The concept of quality of life has been around for many decades, but it has only recently been applied to health care. Patient-determined health-related quality of life (HRQL) is now accepted as a potential outcome measure and is used in both randomized clinical trials and in health services research. HRQL and its separate components can be helpful in documenting both positive and negative treatment effects for the patient.

HRQL represents a multidimensional concept that refers to a person's total well-being. Most people agree that it encompasses three components — physical, social and emotional — and one item assessing the global quality of life. Other dimensions, such as cognitive and intimacy/sexual functioning, may also be measured, depending on the nature of the trial and its intervention. Quality-adjusted life years (QALY), a global measure of patient preferences, is rarely used in clinical trials and will not be discussed here.

Critics of the HRQL concept point to the lack of a consensus definition of quality of life. They also consider that the various diverse HRQL measures are subjective and, therefore, question the validity of any findings. They also criticize the sensitivity of the measures and whether they can be used to detect effects of intervention that are clearly important.

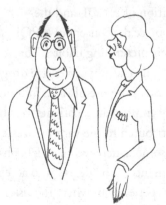

— WE MUST HAVE AN OBJECTIVE MEASURE OF SATISFACTION. SO MANY MISGUIDED PEOPLE THINK THEY'RE REALLY HAPPY.

What is the usefulness of quality of life assessments?

Quality of life measures can sometimes produce unexpected results. A study evaluated the effects of antihypertensive drug treatment on various aspects of well-being using interviews with the patients themselves, their spouses or "significant" others, and their physicians.[2] The physicians reported no noticeable change in their patients' well-being, as blood pressure was usually controlled and the patients had not complained. In contrast, three-quarters of the spouses had noted moderate to severe deterioration in the patients' behaviors and attitudes. Adverse effects noted were a decline in energy and general activity, preoccupation with illness, changes in mood and memory, and reduced libido. Some patients admitted certain negative effects of treatment. In general, the effects of treatment on a person's well-being are best assessed by the patients themselves, or someone who knows them well, rather than by their physician.

The perceptions — "How do you rank your health?" and "How do you rank your well-being?" — are summary global measures that only the patient can address. They represent integrated responses to the overall positive and negative effects of a treatment. For example, does the pain relief of an anti-anginal drug outweigh the potential adverse effects of cold feet, fatigue or headache?

Assessment of HRQL is important not only in the treatment of chronic disorders, where one wants to avoid making symptoms worse, but also in life-threatening conditions, where the patient may regard the quality of life to be as important, or even more important, than the quantity of life. It is always essential that the patient should participate in treatment choice decisions.

Despite a lack of consensus on the definition of HRQL and the importance of measured changes, clinicians embrace the concept of HRQL and allow results from clinical trials to influence their prescribing habits. For example, a heavily promoted report[1] comparing three antihypertensive drugs in terms of HRQL contributed to a marked increase in the use of ACE inhibitors for hypertension. Since hypertension is often asymptomatic, patients may be unwilling to accept the many adverse effects attributed to the various classes of antihypertensive compounds — impotence, insomnia, depression, cough, obstipation, dry mouth and reduced exercise performance. The decision to accept these problems may be most difficult in mild hypertension, where the risk for serious hypertensive complications is small for the individual patient.

Even intermittent conditions such as migraine headaches may affect a patient's HRQL, even between symptomatic attacks. For example, the uncertainty of when or where the next migraine headache may occur may cause patients to change their daily routine and avoid meetings, social gatherings, and travel. Despite the fact that HRQL issues such as this can greatly impact family and friends, they can be difficult to identify. Effective treatment of acute migraine not only can reduce the severity of the headaches themselves, but also can improve quality of life between attacks.

HRQL is equally important in life-threatening conditions such as cancers. Physicians, particularly in the past, often assumed that every effort should be made to extend life even if the odds of a successful outcome were small. This attitude has changed in recent years, and many patients with advanced cancers are now pressing for less toxic treatments and wish to spend more time at home. There has been a shift in the management of the cancer patient, with a focus now on improving the quality of life as well as survival.

What are the methodological challenges?

Inclusion of HRQL assessments in clinical trials presents a special challenge. This may, in part, explain why the FDA has yet to approve an investigational drug based on improvements in HRQL. One issue is that of multiple testing. The standardized questionnaires used to assess HRQL have numerous questions covering several domains. Analysis of individual questions, or subscales, would only increase the likelihood of obtaining a number of statistically significant differences due to the play of chance alone. On the other hand, combining a large number of questions into a single HRQL index may result in the loss of information. This is similar to combining all blood chemistry values into a single overall laboratory index. A reasonable compromise is to limit the number of questions to those relevant to the disease and expected treatment effect and to combine only those that are related.

Another difficulty with most HRQL measures is that they may be influenced by non-health related factors such as marital problems or a change in employment. It is easy to see how these can affect a person's emotional status, sleep, general well-being and even leisure-time activities. Although these issues can confound the assessment of HRQL, randomized trials should yield similar frequencies of these factors across study groups.

Finally, in reading reports from a trial examining HRQL, it is important to ensure that the scientific question was prespecified. In a large number of reported trials, quality of life measures have been deficient on this point.

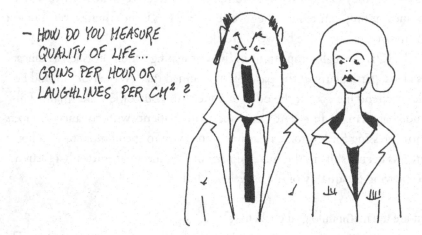

— HOW DO YOU MEASURE
QUALITY OF LIFE...
GRINS PER HOUR OR
LAUGHLINES PER CM² ?

Key Points

- ☞ Health related quality of life (HRQL) is a multidimensional concept referring to a person's total well-being.
- ☞ It encompasses three components — physical, social and emotional — and one item assessing global quality of life.
- ☞ It is clinically relevant in most clinical conditions.
- ☞ An individual's HRQL is described more fully the greater the number of items on the questionnaire.
- ☞ There is a methodological conflict between the number of questionnaire items and hypothesis testing.

"Don't throw the baby out with the bath water"

Chapter 13

What is the value of biologic markers in drug evaluation?

Clinical trials evaluating whether a new treatment reduces morbidity and/or mortality often follow large populations for years. Since such projects require a major financial commitment, it is tempting to look for ways to reduce costs. The use of disease markers is appealing since it is cost saving.

Decades ago, biologic measures purportedly associated with disease status or progression (known collectively as "surrogate endpoints" or "biologic markers,") were proposed as substitutes for morbid or fatal events in clinical trial designs. According to an official in a drug regulatory agency,[6] "a surrogate endpoint of a clinical trial is a laboratory measurement or a physical sign used as a substitute for a clinically useful endpoint that measures directly how a patient feels, functions or survives." The underlying clinical and regulatory assumptions are that improvement in a surrogate benefits the patient clinically and is equivalent to reducing the rate of non-fatal events or mortality. The bridge between the surrogate and the clinical event of interest is critical. Experience so far has been disappointing.[1,3]

What went wrong?
Ventricular extrasystoles on the electrocardiogram, serum cholesterol, and bone density serve as examples of surrogate endpoints. The presence of ventricular extrasystoles in coronary patients is associated with higher mortality and sudden death, elevated levels of serum cholesterol are related to the risk of acute myocardial infarction and premature death, and low bone density is linked to the risk of fractures. In principle, treatment that reduces the frequency of ventricular extrasystoles, reduces serum cholesterol, or increases bone density should reduce morbidity and mortality, *if* the links between the surrogates and outcome(s) are strong, and *if* the surrogate is in the causal pathway. Of course, trials using

surrogate outcomes have a smaller sample size than conventional morbidity/mortality studies, so the available information regarding intervention safety is compromised. There are few good surrogate markers of drug safety. Increases in liver function tests predict liver damage or failure and QT prolongation on the electrocardiogram is associated with higher risks of serious ventricular arrhythmias and sudden cardiac death.

The widespread presumption that premature ventricular extrasystoles might cause sudden cardiac death served as the basis for the design of the Cardiac Arrhythmia Suppression Trial (CAST), sponsored by the National Heart, Lung, and Blood Institute. The primary objective of CAST was to determine whether the use of specific drugs to reduce ventricular extrasystoles in survivors of an acute myocardial infarction also reduced the risk of sudden cardiac death.[2] Eligible subjects were treated with one of three antiarrhythmic agents or a corresponding placebo. All three agents showed the anticipated substantial reduction of ventricular extrasystoles on 24-hour ambulatory ECG monitoring. Unfortunately, this effect did not translate into a reduction of sudden death. Due to an excess number of sudden cardiac deaths in those treated with flecainide (Tambocor) and encainide (Enkaid), CAST was terminated early, after an average of only 10 months of follow-up and enrollment of 1,727 subjects. Thirty-three of 730 participants treated with flecainide or encainide (4.5%) died or suffered a cardiac arrest compared to nine of 725 in the placebo group (1.2%). Although antiarrhythmic treatment successfully reduced the number of ventricular extrasystoles as anticipated, it unexpectedly increased the risk of dying. Clearly, the reduction of ventricular extrasystoles was not a good surrogate of treatment benefit to the patient.

The Heart and Estrogen/progestin Replacement Study (HERS) was designed to determine whether hormone replacement therapy, known to lower LDL cholesterol and raise HDL cholesterol, would reduce the risk of coronary events. A fixed combination of conjugated estrogen (Premarin) and medroxy-progesterone (Provera) was evaluated in a placebo-controlled, long-term trial of about 2,800 postmenopausal women with established coronary heart disease. Based on the observed net mean reduction in LDL cholesterol (11%) and mean increase in HDL cholesterol (10%) at one year and the known statistical associations between mean changes in LDL and HDL cholesterol and risk of coronary events, one would have predicted a treatment benefit of approximately 30%. Surprisingly, however, there was no overall difference in coronary events between the hormone group and the controls in HERS.[4] In the first year, there was even a trend towards an excess number of fatal and non-fatal coronary events in women receiving active therapy. This study shows that drugs may have many different mechanisms of action and that relying on a single surrogate (improved lipid profile) can be very misleading.

The inverse association between bone density and bone fractures is another example of the disparity between theory and reality. Reduced bone density is associated with an increased risk of fractures. This represents a significant health problem among the growing number of elderly individuals, especially women. Hip and vertebral fractures cause substantial suffering and contribute to escalating health-care costs. Sodium fluoride is an inexpensive, generic compound known to stimulate bone formation. A clinical trial from the Mayo

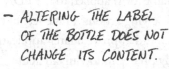

— ALTERING THE LABEL OF THE BOTTLE DOES NOT CHANGE ITS CONTENT.

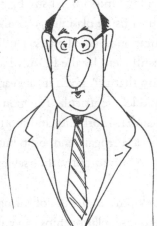

clinic confirmed that sodium fluoride significantly increased bone density.[5] The findings initially suggested that the investigators had discovered a cost-effective method of preventing fractures. In a 3-year follow-up study, bone density and the incidence of fractures were determined. The extended study confirmed the positive effect of sodium fluoride on bone density. Unfortunately, the analyses also showed a three-fold increase in the number of non-vertebral fractures in the sodium fluoride group compared to the placebo group; the incidence of vertebral fractures was 30% higher in the active treatment group than in the controls. The explanation appears to be that sodium fluoride actually promotes the formation of brittle bones.

Are there any reliable surrogate markers?

The amount of virus in the blood of Human Immunodeficiency Virus (HIV)-infected patients — viral load — has proven to be useful for predicting time to AIDS onset and prognosis. Although the use of viral load led to a faster regulatory approval and marketing of new HIV drugs, its value as a surrogate marker has not lived up to the high expectations.

Left ventricular dysfunction following an acute myocardial infarction is associated with premature mortality. A primary objective of treatment in the acute phase of a myocardial infarction is to limit heart muscle damage. Thrombolytic therapy limits infarct size by dissolving the coronary thrombus. One manufacturer of tissue plasminogen activator (tPA) applied to the FDA for approval of the compound based on its clot-dissolving action. This effect of tPA was considered insufficient by the FDA, which did approve a later application after demonstration that tPA given in the early phases following an acute infarction improved left ventricular function. Ventricular function is more closely related to cardiac morbidity and mortality than clot lysis. The FDA rejected clot lysis as a surrogate endpoint, but accepted left ventricular function as a surrogate outcome for mortality, thus saving time, money, and possibly human lives.

In drug development, the use of surrogate markers may be appropriate. Studies of dose-response relationships can guide manufacturers in decisions about future event trials. In serious conditions, the use of a surrogate outcome might be justified for conditional approval of a drug, while proper outcome trials are being conducted.

Key Points

- Treatment effects on biologic markers may or may not reflect effects on clinical events.
- Uncertainties about surrogate markers being good substitutes undermine their value.
- Drugs have multiple mechanisms of action; the biologic marker typically focuses on just one of them.
- There are only a few good markers for drug safety.

"In theory, there is no difference between theory and practice, in practice there is"

(Y. Berra)

Chapter 14

How are adverse drug reactions measured?

There is no perfectly safe drug. All drugs result in some adverse effects. Their severity ranges from mild symptoms to serious health events. An article in *JAMA*[7] reported that the number of fatal adverse drug reactions among U.S. hospital patients approximates 100,000/year, making this type of fatality the fifth leading cause of death. A subsequent report claimed that the total number might be even higher.[6] The challenge is to reduce this staggering number. A study conducted in the U.K. concluded that as many as 6.5% of all hospital admissions were related to an ADR.[8] Most of these ADRs were either definitely or possibly avoidable.

How are adverse effects quantified?

Decisions about treatment should always involve weighing potential treatment benefits against potential risks. In this context, "risk" connotes anything negative associated with a treatment. Although risk refers primarily to direct adverse effects (symptoms) or events, it also includes indirect treatment effects such as labeling a person as diseased or restricting aspects of his or her activities of daily living. Hence, it is important to determine the overall risk burden when making treatment decisions. The costs to society are discussed in Chapter 24.

Measuring the many dimensions of adverse effects is a problem. When reviewing a clinical trial report, clinicians should be aware of several issues concerning the adverse effect profile of a drug. The first occurrence of a specific adverse effect is usually fairly obvious to the patient or physician and is commonly presented as a cumulative percentage at certain time points, or at the end of the trial. Cumulative percentages, however, do not reflect two other important dimensions of adverse effects — their severity and persistence. Patients are typically asked to report how they perceived the severity of an adverse effect, using a scale — severe, moderate or mild. Adverse effects may also be classified by investigators as "severe" (necessitating discontinuation of treatment), "moderate" (leading to dose reductions) or "mild" (no change in treatment or dosing). Persistence of particular adverse effects is difficult to capture and report, especially when symptoms vary in severity.

Other problems relate to lack of definitions for many symptoms such as nausea, fatigue and insomnia. In practice, validating or verifying these symptoms is impossible, since they are self-reported. This fact does in no way limited their importance. The frequency of adverse effect recording is also a factor to consider. The number of adverse events reported depends, in large part, on how often this information is collected. Finally, elicited responses ("Have you had any headaches since the last visit?") yield higher frequencies than open-ended questions ("Since the last visit, have you had any problems with your study medication?").

Clinical trials that are conducted for FDA regulatory purposes require that unanticipated symptoms and complications be classified according to "relatedness." Investigators must judge whether such adverse events are related, possible related, unlikely related or unrelated to the study medication. Since these judgments are highly subjective, they are of limited value, particularly in clinical trials that do not employ a double-blind design.

What are the challenges in attributing causation?
It is sometimes difficult to decide what constitutes a true adverse drug effect. As an extreme example, a patient in a diabetes trial of glycemic control was involved in a car accident that caused the death of the other driver. Is it possible that the accident could have been caused by the study subject suffering a hypoglycemic attack? Should this fatality be classified as an adverse effect and the consequence of tight control of blood sugar?

If the universe of all possible adverse effects were known at the outset, data collection would be fairly straightforward. The challenge is capturing unanticipated adverse drug effects. After all, the general practitioner may not link his/her sedative prescription to a patient's hip fracture[12] and the urologist may overlook the association between the estrogen-treated patient with prostate cancer and his admission for an acute myocardial infarction or stroke. Many drugs have unexpected adverse effects that do not surface until years after their introduction. Thiazide diuretics had been on the market for two decades before their association with impotence was reported. The link between ACE inhibitors and coughing was discovered years after these agents were introduced commercially.

One difficulty arises when the study drug and the treated condition cause the same complication. The most severe adverse reaction induced by the antiarrhythmic agents in the Cardiac Arrhythmia Suppression Trial was sudden cardiac death, the very complication these agents were supposed to prevent! Another example is suicide, which is a possible consequence of depression, but is also associated with the use of anti-depressant medications.[4]

The FDA system for reporting adverse experiences during a clinical trial is designed to uncover unknown or unexpected associations. All serious events such as deaths and hospitalizations must be reported within seven days, regardless of whether or not they are believed to be caused by the study medication. The effectiveness of this system is debatable. One disadvantage of the FDA reporting requirements is that it results in enormous flow of data and a long list

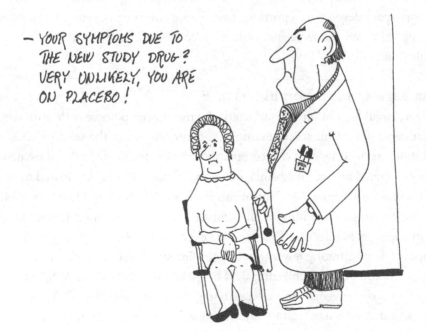

of potential adverse effects that might or might not be due to a drug. Assessing causality can also be difficult, and this is where the randomized, placebo-controlled trial is valuable. The difference in the incidence between the groups receiving active treatment and placebo represents the best estimate of true drug-induced adverse effects.

How completely are adverse drug reactions reported in the literature?

There are no universally accepted methods for reporting adverse effects in trial publications. Similar trial designs employ different approaches to measuring and reporting drug adverse effects. Ioannidis and Lau[5] reviewed the reporting of adverse effects in 192 large clinical trials from seven therapeutic areas. The reporting was considered adequate in only 39% of the articles. Laboratory abnormalities were only presented in approximately a quarter of the publications; about half of them did not even mention any presence of treatment-induced abnormalities. Information on the number of enrolled patients who terminated treatment was missing in a quarter of the papers; the reasons for treatment termi-nation were presented for only 46% of the cases reporting this information. The journal space devoted to reporting adverse drug effects was less than half a page, or approximately the same space taken up by the list of authors and their affiliations.

Can drug safety be a primary trial outcome?

Clinical trials are not often conducted with the primary purpose of determining treatment safety. One recent example is an integral part of the selective COX-2 inhibitor story. It was discovered early during drug development that these newer 'coxibs' offered no overall advantage in terms of pain relief, as compared to the traditional non-steroidal anti-inflammatory drugs (NSAIDs), but that they might be less irritating to the lining of the stomach. To provide a competitive edge, the manufacturers of rofecoxib (Vioxx) and celecoxib (Celebrex) initiated trials, in hopes of demonstrating fewer serious gastrointestinal (GI) complications (perforations, ulcers and bleedings). The trials, VIGOR[1] and CLASS,[9] were set up to compare rofecoxib and celecoxib to generic, non-selective NSAIDs. VIGOR showed a significant reduction in serious GI events, but at the expense of an offsetting increase in major vascular events. CLASS also reported a GI benefit, but only after redefining the study outcome *post-hoc* and excluding the data from the second 6 months of the one-year trial. The increase in major thrombotic events (mainly acute myocardial infarction) with the coxibs, a recognized class effect, was confirmed in 2004 in two placebo-controlled trials in patients with colon polyps.[2,10] The manufacturer of rofecoxib decided on a voluntary recall of the drug from the market, whereas the manufacturer of celecoxib did not.

Although treatment safety is rarely the main focus of a clinical trial, safety trials are fairly common in the cancer field. These are typically conducted to determine which of two treatments is least harmful.

Are you reporting observed adverse drug reactions for your practice?

Although FDA's major source for identifying safety problems post-marketing is the Adverse Event Reporting System (AERS), cooperation from practicing clinicians and patients is of great importance. MedWatch, a passive, largely outdated voluntary system provides valuable safety information from these sources in spite of massive underreporting, estimated to be in the range of 90-99%.[11] The major value of MedWatch relates to the detection of rare, unexpected serious drug reactions. More proactive approaches for the early detection of harmful drug effects in the marketplace have been proposed.[3]

Key Points

- All drugs cause some adverse effects.
- These adverse effects have several dimensions — frequency, severity and persistence.
- It is difficult to assign causality when the drug and the treated condition produce the same effects.
- Trial publications typically give inadequate attention to drug safety.

"Better to be safe than sorry"

Chapter 15

How representative are study subjects in clinical trials?

Study subjects agreeing to participate in clinical trials *rarely* constitute a representative sample of patients in the general population who have the condition under study.

The trial protocol usually calls for exclusion of patients with the poorest prognosis. Thus, those with concomitant diseases affecting prognosis, those with advanced stages of the condition and elderly individuals are usually excluded from participation. The desire for a "clean" experiment without contamination by therapies or conditions other than the one(s) under study comes at the expense of having the ability to extrapolate trial findings to all patients with the condition under study. As a result, trial conclusions may over- or under-estimate true drug effects. Safety problems are usually underestimated. Clinicians often need to judge the value of a treatment, based on incomplete information.

Trial participation in itself may also influence trial results. Study subjects usually receive special attention and optimal care, including close monitoring. Special tests and procedures that are not part of regular care may uncover complications or other conditions, leading to earlier intervention. Thus, mere participation in a trial may have favorable health effects. These effects, however, ought to be the same in the intervention and control groups.

Exclusion of the sickest patients and the possible health benefits of trial participation also have implications for statistical power. The event or complication rates are likely to be lower than the estimates for an unselected patient population, thus reducing statistical power for the trial. If the sample size is not increased accordingly, the trial could be an inadequate test of the intervention.

How selective are study populations?

A group of Finnish investigators conducted a retrospective chart review.[2] The typical eligibility criteria for clinical trials of patients with gastric ulcer were applied to 400 patients hospitalized with the diagnosis of gastric ulcer. Only 29% of the patients met the eligibility criteria and almost all deaths and serious complications such as gastric bleeding, perforation and stenosis during the first five to seven years occurred among those patients who would have been ineligible. Clearly, the testing of H_2 - blockers or other compounds for the prevention of long-term complications of gastric ulcer in low-risk patients should not be generalized to the entire ulcer population.

Two further examples illustrate the selective nature of clinical trial populations. A review of subjects enrolled in trials of NSAIDs showed that only 2.1% were 65 years of age or older, in spite of the fact that these drugs are more commonly used in the elderly.[4]

In patients who survive a myocardial infarction and are discharged from hospital, one-year mortality is approximately 7-9%. However, many controlled trials have reported a placebo group mortality of just 3-4%. The explanation is

— THE TRIAL WAS SO EXCLUSIVE THAT NO ONE WAS EVER RANDOMIZED.

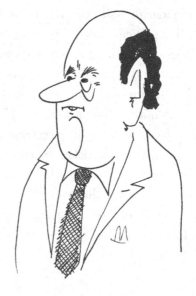

simple — the high-risk patients are often excluded in the clinical studies. As a consequence, secondary prevention trials in infarction patients must be large, in order to demonstrate risk reductions of the magnitude of 20-25%.

How may selection bias affect trial findings?

Exclusion of high-risk patients in clinical trials has other ramifications. Several post myocardial infarction studies that evaluated prophylactic beta-blocker therapy included patients with a broader spectrum of risk. Contrary to what one would expect, these trials showed that the benefits of beta-blockade were more pronounced in patients with complicated infarcts (and no contraindications to beta-blocker therapy) than in patients with uncomplicated infarcts.[1] By excluding high-risk patients, beneficial effects may be missed.

Selection bias may also increase the chances of finding favorable treatment effects. Study subjects typically have above-average education, as well as a personal interest in the research project. As a consequence, their level of adherence with the study medication is usually high. Additionally, since study subjects are usually free of other conditions and take few if any other medications (*healthy volunteer effect*), the likelihood of drug- drug interactions is small.

A focus on low-risk patients can lead to an underestimation of harmful drug effects and/or a delay in their detection. The development of the selective COX-2 inhibitors serves as a recent example. By conducting small, short-term trials in mostly low-risk subjects, the safety signals pointing to this class of agents causing serious thrombotic events (especially heart attacks) were missed.

According to a Medline search, there were 1,430 randomized clinical trials of calcium channel blockers published between 1990 and 1995.[3] Most of them focused on surrogate outcomes. There was no single large trial conducted during that period to determine whether and to what extent these agents reduce the risks of strokes, heart attacks and heart failure in subjects with hypertension, the major indication for these agents.

Key Points

- Study populations often represent a highly selected sample of people in the general population.
- Exclusion of high-risk patients may lead to an underestimation of harmful effects.
- Exercise caution in extrapolating trial results to individuals not meeting trial entry criteria.

"You can't make a silk purse out of a sow's ear"

Chapter 16

What happened to the study subjects who disappeared from the analysis?

Withdrawal of randomized patients from the primary data analysis of treatment efficacy constitutes one of the major potential sources of bias in clinical trials. This practice of omitting selected patients from the analysis is less common nowadays, but readers should still be aware of it. Withdrawing randomized subjects from the analysis can distort study findings, most often by favoring the group receiving the active or new intervention. Experience has shown that the number of enrolled patients who stop taking their study medication due to adverse effects, lack of anticipated benefit or other reasons can vary substantially, from just a few to up to one-third. Any loss of patients to follow-up should immediately prompt the question "What happened to the participants who disappeared from the analysis?" This problem has been highlighted by regulatory agencies, which now require full accounting of all randomized participants in a trial, as well as specifications about reasons for participant withdrawals.

What are the reasons given?

The following three reasons are typically given for withdrawing randomized study subjects from the analysis.

First, the study subject did not meet the eligibility (inclusion/exclusion) criteria. This explanation is particularly troublesome if the decision to withdraw is made after the study subject has started or, worse, has completed the trial. Most trials have at least a few such "protocol violators." Since they were already randomized, their exclusion jeopardizes the baseline comparability of study groups established by randomization. If the number of such protocol violators is high, one has to question the overall quality of the trial and its execution. If these violators are retained in the final analysis, the integrity of the study is preserved.

Second, since study subjects who do not take their assigned medications as intended cannot benefit from treatment, they are withdrawn for the analysis. There are several reasons why patients do not take their pills, including the development of adverse effects or lack of anticipated treatment benefit. If one were to withdraw from the analysis all study subjects who suffered adverse drug effects, some of which may be serious, and report only on those who tolerated the drug, the final conclusions would be misleading. Also, actively treated study subjects who develop adverse drug effects are often sicker than other participants. Omitting them could, therefore, also undermine group comparability. The best way to avoid analytic pitfalls is to include all randomized study subjects in the primary analysis according to their originally assigned treatment groups. This approach is called the *intention-to-treat analysis.*

Third, subjects are sometimes withdrawn because they have missing data. Every trial has its share of missing values, perhaps due to missed clinic visits or human error. Missing data is no justification for omitting a subject from the analysis, because the reason why data are missing may be treatment-related. The golden rule is that all randomized patients should be followed until the conclusion of a trial and presented in the primary analysis. As much information as possible should be collected and presented on subjects withdrawing from a trial.

— INTERPOL HAS ISSUED WARRANTS FOR 29 SUBJECTS WHO DISAPPEARED FROM A CLINICAL TRIAL.

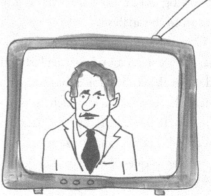

How do withdrawals affect reported findings?

The Anturane Reinfarction Trial (ART) represents a striking example of how withdrawal of randomized study subjects can favorably influence reported trial results.[1] The FDA even took the unusual step of criticizing the sponsor in an article published in the New England Journal of Medicine.[5] The objective of ART was to determine whether the platelet-active drug sulfinpyrazone (Anturane) improved prognosis over a two-year period among survivors of acute myocardial infarction. One criticism focused on the withdrawal of 71 of the 1,629 randomized study subjects from the analysis. It was claimed that these 71 participants did not meet the study eligibility criteria. Of the withdrawals, 38 had been randomized to the sulfinpyrazone group and 33 had been assigned to the placebo group -- hardly a difference that would warrant attention. However, 10 of the 38 (26.3%) withdrawn sulfinpyrazone patients died versus only four of the 33 (12.1%) withdrawn placebo participants. Many reasons for withdrawal from analysis in ART were subjective and were not applied until after the study subjects had completed the trial or had died! The difference in the number of deaths among study subjects withdrawn from the analysis contributed to the reported statistically significant mortality results favoring sulfinpyrazone.

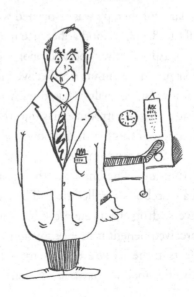

— DARN, THIS TRIAL WOULD BE SIGNIFICANT IF I COULD JUST EXCLUDE ONE MORE EVENT FROM THE TREATMENT GROUP.

The Coronary Drug Project (CDP) compared the effects of several lipid-lowering regimens versus placebo on all-cause mortality in patients with a history of myocardial infarction. The 5-year mortality in one of the active groups (clofibrate) was 20.0% compared to 20.9% in the placebo group. Since drug adherence is important in a prophylactic trial of this kind, subgroup analyses were conducted based on reported level of drug adherence.[2] Good compliers were compared to poor compliers in the clofibrate group. When the results showed a 5-year mortality of 15.0% among the good compliers and 24.6% among the poor compliers, everything seemed to make sense. Maybe CDP would have had a positive outcome if all subjects in the clofibrate group had faithfully taken their study medication? However, analysis by level of adherence in the placebo group also revealed greater survival among the good vs. the poor compliers (5-year mortality of 15.1% versus 28.2%, respectively). In a similar analysis of drug adherence in heart failure patients, mortality was approximately 35% lower among good adherers compared to poor adherers.[3] Taken at face value, this makes sense for a drug with superior efficacy. Unfortunately, this observation was true for both actively treated patients and those taking placebo. A recent meta-analysis of 21 trials concluded that good adherence to placebo was associated with lower mortality (OR = 0.56, 95% CI 0.43 to 0.63) and that good adherence to harmful therapy was associated with increased mortality (OR = 2.40, 95% CI 1.04 to 8.11).[4] Good adherence may be a marker for overall healthy behavior.

Apparently, good and poor compliers are different in a number of ways and their prognosis differs irrespective of treatment received. Withdrawing patients from statistical analysis based on whether or not they took their assigned treatment can introduce bias into the study conclusions. The extent and direction of this bias is unknown.

Some randomized studies follow subjects until they stop taking their study medication. The impact of this approach is likely to favor the active medication in a placebo-controlled trial. The reasons for stopping treatment are different -- adverse drug effects are more common in the active group, while lack of perceived benefit is more common among controls. Those who have adverse effects in the active group are more likely to be at high risk. Excluding them from the analysis may bias the results. Limiting the analysis to compliant subjects is referred to as "*analysis by treatment administered.*" Such analysis should never replace intention-to-treat analyses.

Key Points

o═ Group comparability achieved through randomization may be compromised by withdrawing randomized subjects.

o═ Withdrawing randomized subjects from the analysis may distort trial results.

o═ The intention-to-treat approach trumps the "per treatment administered" approach.

"Love and a cough cannot be hid"

Chapter 17

How reliable are active-control trials?

We should all be grateful to the pharmaceutical industry for developing the large number of beneficial drugs that are available today. For most conditions, physicians have many treatment choices. Although there have been several 'blockbuster' drugs that have completely changed the management of a particular disease, they are the exception. Major breakthroughs in pharmacological treatment of a disease come along only once in a while and most drugs produced by pharmaceutical companies today offer limited improvement, in terms of efficacy or tolerability over what is already available. This desire for innovation, even if it is only incremental, is driven by the limited patent life of a product. Once the patent on a 'branded' drug has expired, it becomes 'generic' and can be produced by several manufacturers with few regulatory hurdles. With the protection from competition removed, the price of the drug to the consumer falls, as does the profit to the manufacturer. Consequently, there is a continual need for pharmaceutical companies to develop new patented drugs, even if they offer no or minor advances over existing ones. Most new drugs introduced today fall into this category. Evaluating a new drug for an indication for which there already are many recognized treatment alternatives introduces a different sort of challenge. Since use of a placebo may not be ethical, the new drug has to be compared to one of the drugs accepted as safe and efficacious.

Comparative, or active-control trials introduce new issues of design, conduct, analysis and interpretation. In general, placebo-controlled trials have a more predictable outcome than comparative trials. One overriding question should be asked about all active-control trials: Was the comparison meaningful and fair?

Who sponsored the trial?

In a review of all active-control trials of second-generation antipsychotic drugs for the treatment of schizophrenia, 33 of the 42 trials were sponsored by pharmaceutical companies.[8] While this was not surprising, since non-commercial institutions lack incentives to conduct such trials, it was disturbing that 90% of the studies favored the sponsors' products. Of the nine head-to-head comparisons of olanzapine (Zyprexa) and risperidone (Risperdal), the five trials sponsored by the manufacturer of olanzapine all favored its agent, while three of the four sponsored by the manufacturer of risperidone did the same. It seems likely that the two sponsors designed the trials to highlight the benefits of their own products, or alternatively, to underestimate the benefits of the comparator.

For clinical, ethical and scientific reasons, active-control trials should compare new drugs to *optimal* treatments that are generally available. Patients should never be exposed to sub-standard care.[18] Marketing considerations should not be the primary factor when selecting a comparator drug. Clinically, we want to know whether a new treatment offers any advantages over existing ones and what these advantages might be. Always be on the alert when evaluating the results of a commercially sponsored active-control trial and ask the following questions:

Was selection of the active-control fair?

In evaluating an antihypertensive drug, the optimal comparator should be a low-dose diuretic, which has proven to be highly beneficial in reducing all vascular complications of hypertension, is fairly safe when properly used, and is very inexpensive.[14] Since showing superiority over, or even equality with, a generic diuretic is difficult, a manufacturer of a novel class of antihypertensive agents or of a new member of an established class (so-called 'me-too' drugs) may tip the balance in favor of its drug[15] In LIFE[2] and in ASCOT,[3] losartan (Cozaar) and amlodipine (Norvasc) were compared to atenolol given once daily. Atenolol is clearly inferior to thiazide diuretics[14] and appears to be the least effective beta-blocker for the treatment of hypertension[1,12] and for secondary prevention post-infarction.[6] A once-daily regimen of atenolol may not provide adequate blood pressure control over 24 hours. LIFE and ASCOT, though positive for losartan and amlodipine, were therefore fairly uninformative with regard to how hypertensive patients should best be treated.[15]

Was the dose of the comparative drug appropriate?

As the patent for the proton-pump inhibitor omeprazole (Losec) was about to expire, the manufacturer introduced esomeprazole (Nexium), the more potent isomer of the racemic omeprazole. The approved and recommended daily dose of omeprazole is 20 mg. The equipotent dose of esomeprazole was estimated to range between 10 and 20 mg daily. In active-control trials in patients with duodenal ulcers, the sponsor chose to compare "double doses" of 20 and 40 mg of esomeprazole with 20 mg of omeprazole. Not surprisingly, esomeprazole came out ahead, but only by a very small margin in terms of "healing rates."[4,11] This small difference was key to an effective marketing campaign, but a fairer study would have compared equipotent doses of the two drugs.

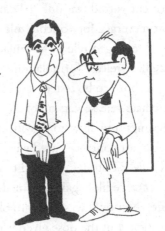

- TOO BAD, OUR NEW DRUG ONLY OFFERS LIMITED ADVANTAGES.
- NO PROBLEM, SKILLFUL MARKETING WILL MAKE IT A BLOCKBUSTER.

In a review of 56 trials evaluating various NSAIDs for the treatment of arthritis, every study reported the sponsor's drug to be either superior (29%) or comparable (71%) to the NSAID used in the control group.[16] In almost half of these trials, the dose of the sponsor's drug was judged to be higher than that of the comparator drug!

Was the approved formulation of the comparative drug used?

In a meta-analysis of trials comparing fluconazole (Diflucan), a new antifungal drug, with amphotericin B in cancer patients, the investigators had a problem.[9] Three of the trials (43% of patients) also included a group of patients treated with nystatin, which is known to be ineffective as a systemic antifungal agent in patients with a low white cell count, a common complication of cancer. The results for the amphotericin B patients were combined with those of the nystatin patients, producing a bias in favor of fluconazole. The trial authors and sponsor declined to provide results broken down by treatment group. In addition, 79% of the active-control patients received an oral formulation of amphotericin B, which is poorly absorbed and only approved for treating fungal infections of the mouth. For systemic infections, it is well known that amphotericin B should be given intravenously.

In a trial of voriconazole (Vfend) by the same sponsor, the amphotericin B-treated patients were neither pre-medicated to minimize toxic reactions nor given fluids and electrolytes to reduce nephrotoxicity.[10] For these reasons, the mean treatment period was only 10 days for the amphotericin group compared to 77 days on average for voriconazole.

Prolonged-release formulations can be administered less frequently than immediate-release formulations. If a new prolonged-release formulation of a drug is about to be tested, it makes sense to use the prolonged rather than the immediate-release version of any comparator. Unfortunately, manufacturers are sometimes unwilling to provide drug supplies to a competitor for a trial which they do not control. Faced with this dilemma, the sponsor and investigators of the COMET study[13] decided to test a prolonged-release formulation of the beta-blocker calvedilol against immediate-release metoprolol in patients with heart failure. Not only was metoprolol in this formulation not approved for this indication, but the dose given was too low. Not surprisingly, calvedilol showed a survival advantage. The question remains… was this observed advantage due to the lower dose of metoprolol, due to its short-acting formulation, or due to a combination of both?

Was the assessment of outcomes appropriate?

Comparing an agent with a long duration of action to one with a short duration can also be challenging. Timolol eye drops are a standard treatment for managing glaucoma. The maximum reduction in intraocular pressure (IOP) occurs after 1-2 hours and then wears off rapidly. Hence, multiple daily applications are required. In contrast, latanoprost is a prostaglandin analog with maximum IOP reduction after 8-12 hours. If the two drugs are to be fairly compared, IOP measurements need to be made at several timepoints over the course of the day. In one study that did compare the two drugs, the timing of the IOP measurements was arranged to favor the newer agent.[17] The sponsor decided to delay the 8:00 a.m. morning dose of the timolol drops until after the 9:00 a.m. IOP measurement. Clearly, any IOP-lowering effect of the timolol dose from the previous evening had worn off by that time.

It takes up to 5 days to achieve the full prophylactic effect of warfarin (Coumadin) for thrombosis prevention. A new anticoagulant, ximelagatran (Exanta) reaches therapeutic concentrations within hours. A short-term trial was designed to compare the two agents in patients undergoing surgery for knee prosthesis. The primary combined outcome was mortality plus thromboembolic events over 7-12 days.[7] The new drug showed a lower combined event rate -- mostly for asymptomatic distal thrombi -- but the FDA appropriately rejected the trial as an unfair comparison, since warfarin had never been approved for short-term use.

How was the treatment effect measured?
When event rates in trials comparing two active interventions are low, it is tempting to try and increase statistical power, in hopes of demonstrating an enhanced treatment effect for the new agent as compared to the control drug. Consequently, composite outcomes are often used in active-control trials (Chapter 18). To increase the overall event rate, mortality and major morbidity events are often combined with less severe conditions, such as number of hospitalizations or occurrence of symptoms. Because these less severe events are usually more frequent, they often make a disproportionate contribution to the composite outcome. Another way to artificially differentiate one new drug from another in a composite outcome trial is to exclude events from the composite that may not be favorably influenced by the new drug.

Heart failure, a major vascular complication, is known to be induced by several classes of drugs such as calcium channel blockers and glitazones, but is often under-emphasized in trials of these drugs. In PROactive, a placebo-controlled trial of pioglitazone in Type 2 diabetes, the reported favorable reduction in the composite primary and secondary vascular endpoints in patients receiving pioglitazone was offset when the unfavorable difference in the number of hospitalized heart failures was considered.[5]

What can be done about sponsor bias?

The lack of clear scientific and regulatory guidelines for active-control trials contributes to the problem of *sponsor bias*. We need to ensure independence in the design, conduct, analysis and reporting of these trials. One suggestion would be for the sponsors to make the trial protocols public, preferably by linking them to clinical trial registries. Regulatory authorities and the local Institutional Review Boards charged with protecting research subjects should not accept trial protocols with unfair comparisons. Medical journals should pay more attention to this issue and should not publish results from trials with design bias. Unfortunately, this issue has not yet received the attention it needs and deserves.

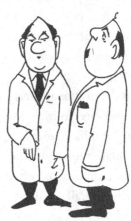

— THE UNEXPECTED RESULTS WERE
FAVORABLE TO THE TRIAL SPONSOR.
— WHAT A COINCIDENCE !

Key Points

- For a comparative trial to be informative, the comparison must be fair.
- The majority of industry sponsored trials favor the sponsors' drugs.
- Determination of fairness is critical in the evaluation of active-control trials.
- Strict scientific and regulatory guidelines are needed for active-control trials.

"There are tricks in every trade"

Chapter 18

How informative are composite outcomes?

During the past decade, a growing number of clinical trials have adopted composite outcomes to measure treatment efficacy. This makes sense, since many treatments have multiple effects, favorable and unfavorable. Selecting any single effect as the primary outcome may therefore not reflect the overall impact of the treatment. The cost of large-scale, long-term event trials has also driven this trend. By combining the rates of multiple events, sample size can be reduced, treatment duration shortened, and/or statistical power increased to detect smaller relative treatment differences. This is the upside of composite outcomes. There is, however, a downside.

What is the clinical relevance of composite outcomes?

Combining events of similar severity such as cause-specific mortality, non-fatal myocardial infarction and stroke is generally accepted. In addition, the diagnostic criteria for these events are well defined and can be validated. Problems emerge when events of varying severity are combined. Adding self-reported angina, vascular procedures, and hospitalizations to major cardiovascular events is debatable. Whether a patient is hospitalized or has a costly procedure could be seen as a marker of disease severity, but it could also be influenced by whether the patient has health insurance coverage.

Experience has shown that the more subjective and the least serious events that represent components of a composite outcome are the most likely to respond favorably to treatment, compared to events that are more objective and serious. In MIRACL, more than 3,000 patients with unstable angina or non-Q-wave acute myocardial infarctions were randomized to 80 mg of the lipid-lowering drug atorvastatin or placebo and followed for 16 weeks.[5] The risk of the composite outcome, which included all-cause mortality, non-fatal myocardial infarction, cardiac arrest and hospitalization for recurrent ischemic symptoms, was lower in the statin group, although the p-value was only borderline (0.048).

The overall difference between the active and placebo groups was driven by a 26% reduction in hospitalized angina (p=0.02), which comprised 45% of all events. For the harder outcomes, the treatment group differences were smaller and none reached statistical significance. A recent meta-analyses[1] of 12 statin trials in this population (n = 13,024) confirmed that initiation of statin therapy within two weeks of acute coronary syndrome does not reduce death, recurrent infarction or stroke within four months.

When faced with a composite outcome that is statistically significant, always consider 1) why each individual component was selected and 2) its contribution to the overall outcome. The components of a composite endpoint should make clinical sense. Ideally, the most important components should show individual statistical significance, or very strong and consistent trends.

What if the component benefits differ?

How should one interpret a trial if the composite outcome and three of the four components failed to reach statistical difference, but the fourth component was reduced, with a p-value less than 0.05? Unless the protocol pre-specifies secondary analyses of the individual four components, including adjustment of the significance level for multiple analysis (see Chapter 22), the results should be considered inconclusive.

In LIFE,[2] first-line treatment with the angiotensin receptor blocker losartan (Cozaar) was reported to be more effective than the beta-blocker atenolol (Tenormin) in reducing the composite outcome -- cardiovascular mortality, stroke and acute myocardial infarction (see discussion about atenolol in Chapter 17). The major contributor to the modest 13% reduction in the composite outcome (p = 0.02) was a 25% reduction in stroke risk (p < 0.001). There was no significant decrease in the risk of cardiovascular (CV) mortality or myocardial infarction and, in fact, there were more infarctions in the losartan group. How should these findings be interpreted, regulated and promoted? Would it be fair to conclude that losartan reduced the risk of CV mortality, stroke and myocardial infarction (with the latter trending in the wrong direction)? A more rational conclusion would be to say that compared to atenolol, losartan reduced the risk of stroke, but only if the statistically significant stroke difference remained after adjustment for the multiple comparisons (which it did). This is how the U.S. FDA interpreted the LIFE findings.

Why should the significance level be adjusted for component analysis?

This question is addressed in more detail in Chapter 22. In short, the purpose is to protect against over-interpreting chance findings. A conservative approach is to divide the nominal p-value of 0.05 by the number of comparisons (components). Thus, for a composite outcome involving five components, a p-value of 0.01 would be needed to signify differences between treatment groups. Regrettably, adjustments for multiple comparisons are rarely made in published trials with composite outcomes. Journal editors should be more circumspect regarding this important issue.

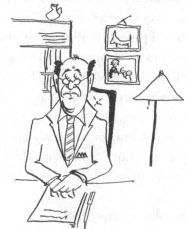

— PATIENTS TAKING THE NEW DRUG HAD FEWER HANGNAILS. UNFORTUNATELY MORE OF THEM DIED!

Can net benefit be determined?

In Chapter 2, we emphasized the importance of considering the benefit-to-harm balance when making treatment decisions. This weighing of favorable and unfavorable treatment effects often relies on different sources and types of information. The use of a composite outcome provides an opportunity to balance diverse treatment effects.

It has not been conclusively documented that glycemic control in patients with Type 2 diabetes leads to a reduction in major cardiovascular events. In the placebo-controlled PROactive trial, the objective was to determine the effect of pioglitazone (Actos) on cardiovascular events.[3] The primary composite outcome included incidence of mortality, nonfatal myocardial infarction, stroke, acute coronary syndrome, revascularizations and amputations. Notably absent was congestive heart failure, a known adverse effect of the glitazones, especially when given in combination with insulin. PROactive failed to show a statistically significant reduction of the primary outcome, but there was a strong favorable trend (RR 0.90, 95% CI 0.80-1.02). The difference for one of the secondary composite outcomes (incidence of mortality, nonfatal myocardial infarction and stroke) reached nominal statistical significance (RR 0.84, 95% CI 0.72-0.98). The numerical reduction for the primary outcome was fifty-eight events and for the secondary outcome fifty-seven events. The authors concluded that pioglitazone improves the cardiovascular outcome in patients with Type-2 diabetes. In the main publication,[3] however, they failed to point out that the drug appears to convey no benefit in diabetic patients treated with statins or beta-blockers. The number of patients in PROactive who were reported to have congestive heart failure was much higher in the pioglitazone group than in the placebo group (281 vs. 198, respectively). The excess of severe heart failure events requiring hospitalization among pioglitazone-treated patients was fifty-six. Thus, the addition of congestive heart failure to the pre-specified primary outcome eliminates the evidence of a meaningful cardiovascular benefit of pioglitazone and rejects the investigators' conclusion. This case illustrates a missed opportunity to assess the net cardiovascular benefit of an intervention.

What is the collective experience?
Freemantle et al.[4] reviewed nine of the leading medical journals during 1997-2001 and found 167 randomized trials with primary composite outcomes. A total of approximately 300,000 patients were enrolled. All-cause mortality was a component in all trials. No statistically significant difference for either the composite outcome or mortality was reported in 63 trials (38%). In 60 trials (36%), the composite outcome showed significant benefit, but not overall mortality. In contrast, both the composite outcome and mortality reached statistical significance in 19 trials (11%). Interestingly, the difference for the composite outcome in six trials (4%) was insignificant while significant for mortality. The

probability of a significant difference more than doubled (OR=2.2) if a subjective component was included.

Can adverse drug reactions be combined?

Absolutely, but this is rarely (if ever) done! The challenges would be similar… the varying clinical relevance of the individual adverse reactions and multiple testing. In an ideal world, the weighted sum of all *unfavorable* drug effects should be compared to the sum of all *favorable* effects. In the absence of established methods for weighing good and bad effects, these decisions are now left to clinicians, many of whom lack the appropriate information and perhaps the skills to make such decisions.

Key Points

o⤜ Always consider the component contributions of a composite outcome.

o⤜ Watch out for "cherry-picked" composite outcomes.

o⤜ There is a noticeable absence of composite safety outcomes.

"The worth of a thing is what it will bring"

Chapter 19

Do changes in biologic markers predict clinical benefit?

The limitations of biologic or surrogate markers in drug evaluation are covered in Chapter 13. In this chapter, we expand the discussion to include the utility of these markers, especially in terms of their treatment-induced effects on patient care and whether findings from the first members of a drug class should be extrapolated to subsequent "me-too" drugs of the same class.

Do surrogate markers predict benefit in individuals?

It has been generally assumed that only patients with hypercholesterolemia or hypertension benefit from lipid-lowering or antihypertensive treatment. Recent trial reports, however, have raised questions about these assumptions.

The Heart Protection Study[1] investigated simvastatin (Zocor) vs. placebo taken over 5 years in 20,500 subjects. The fairly unselected study population included those with normal and abnormal serum lipids, as well as those with and without a history of vascular disease. Convincing subgroup analyses demonstrated that subjects with normal lipids and no vascular history (i.e., those with no indication for statin treatment) benefited the same as those in other subgroups, in terms of relative event reduction. The authors raised the logical question -- Is elevated total or LDL cholesterol in serum a reliable indicator for initiation of lipid-lowering (statin) treatment? Should treatment guidelines and treatment decisions be based only on these measures? Clearly, drugs have multiple mechanisms of action. The challenging question is which mechanism(s) of action should guide regulatory approval and patient care?

The VA-HIT project was designed to determine whether increases in HDL- cholesterol would reduce recurrent coronary events in a long-term, placebo-controlled trial involving more than 2,500 coronary patients. Using multivariate analysis, the investigators determined how much of the observed reduction in coronary events could be explained by the presumed beneficial mechanism of action -- the increase in HDL- cholesterol.[5] The result was surprising -- only 23%! Thus, more than three quarters of the observed benefit was attributable to other mechanisms. This is yet another reminder that drugs have multiple actions. One expected single action (based on a specific surrogate) may not be the major contributor to clinical benefit.

Similar findings seem to apply to the use of antihypertensive treatment. In the PROGRESS project,[3] normotensive patients with a history of cerebrovascular events benefited as much as their hypertensive counterparts. This raises the question... who should start on antihypertensive therapy and when?

Does blood pressure lowering predict clinical benefit?

Blood pressure lowering is one of the most well-known surrogate markers. It is well established that hypertension increases the risks of stroke, acute myocardial infarction and heart failure. A very large number of clinical trials of antihypertensive agents have documented that lowering blood pressure reduces the risk of these vascular complications. But can we conclude that the *entire* benefit of treatment is mediated through blood pressure lowering? Or do antihypertensive agents have meaningful actions that are unrelated to blood pressure lowering? Growing evidence indicates that the latter is the case, so the choice of antihypertensive may be important.

According to many studies, most of the benefit in reducing stroke occurrence is attributable directly to blood pressure lowering. Thus, for stroke prevention, drug selection may be less of an issue. For other vascular events, drug choice is more critical. The ALLHAT study[6] reported that doxazosin (Cardura), an alpha-blocker, doubled the risk of heart failure compared to a diuretic, in spite of similar blood pressure lowering in both groups. The calcium channel blocker amlodipine (Norvasc) increased heart failure risk by 40%, while again yielding equivalent blood pressure reductions in patients receiving amlodipine or a diuretic.[7] These observations confirm that drugs have multiple mechanisms of action and that reliance on just one as a surrogate marker is misguided. These non-blood pressure-mediated actions, which are not yet completely understood, can add to or detract from the benefit of blood pressure lowering *per se*.

Should changes in a surrogate marker be extrapolated within a drug class?

Favorable changes in a surrogate marker are sometimes insufficient to recommend full approval and widespread use of the first drug of a particular class. Clinicians and regulatory agencies prefer to see trial evidence of event reductions. When simvastatin (Zocor) was shown to reduce total and LDL-cholesterol, the FDA approved the drug, but asked for outcome trials. When the first large simvastatin trial, 4S,[6] showed a convincing reduction in all-cause mortality in coronary patients, use of the drug increased markedly. It is appropriate that the clinical criteria for accepting the first drug of a class are the

most stringent. Should later drugs of the same class, the typical "me-too" drugs, be held to the same standard, or would it suffice to show a similar reduction in total and LDL-cholesterol? Experience tells us that the answers are "yes" and "no," respectively.

Cerivastatin (Baycol) was introduced as a potent lipid-lowering agent, and promoted as "another statin." Many were led to believe that it was interchangeable with the other approved statins, which had very positive event and safety data. By lowering the cost of the drug compared to the other brand-name statins, the manufacturer of cerivastatin succeeded in gaining modest market share. However, cerivastatin had harmful non-cholesterol-lowering actions that were never properly reported.[4] It caused a higher risk of rhabdomyo-lysis than the other statins, especially in combination with gemfibrozil (Lopid).[2] Eventually, the drug was removed from the market. This story is just another reminder that drugs have multiple actions and that similarity in one mechanism of action does not mean interchangeability. All members of a drug class ought to be subjected to strict regulatory oversight prior to approval. Evidence of overall health benefits and safety cannot be determined with certainty by investigating surrogate markers.

Key Points
- Biologic markers are imperfect measures in predicting drug benefit or harm.
- Surrogate efficacy should not form the basis for determining class effects.

"A substitute shines brightly as a King until a King be by"
(W. Shakespeare in "The Merchant of Venice")

Chapter 20

How trustworthy are the authors?

The ultimate goal of research is to find true answers to challenging questions. Most scientists share this goal, recognizing that the outcomes of research projects are unpredictable in terms of direction and magnitude. Unfortunately, uncertainty about the outcome of a trial may create conflicts for those with vested or self-serving interests, whether they be financial or scientific. Authors must take full responsibility for their published articles, even if the trials are designed and conducted by a for-profit sponsor.

One key factor contributing to this potential bias relates to the authors of scientific articles, who typically exercise total control over what is reported. Some are tempted to present their results by over-interpreting the good news and/or by downplaying the bad news. Adding a positive spin to study findings has certain advantages. It increases the likelihood of getting the article published in a reputable journal, leads to peer recognition, invitations to conferences and academic promotions, and brings more funding opportunities from industry sponsors.

These potential conflicts of interest are well recognized by medical journal editors, who have taken actions to deal with them. Simple disclosure is easy, but this does not preclude favorable spinning of trial results.

What do journals do?

In 1984, the New England Journal of Medicine was the first medical journal to require authors of original articles to disclose potential conflicts of interest. This requirement was later expanded to writers of editorials. Initially, compliance with this policy was not very strict. Even the *NEJM* admitted failure to follow its own guidance for eighteen review articles.[1]

The rules are getting even more stringent. They now apply to all co-authors and have been broadened to include journal reviewers. Disclosure of potential conflicts is now part of funding decisions at the National Institutes of Health and also contributes to decisions about who can serve on FDA Advisory

Committees. It has been proposed that disclosure itself may affect study credibility.[3] First, after a conflict of interest is disclosed, the person may feel less of an obligation to exercise "balance" (so-called "moral licensing"). Second, the person making a disclosure could assume that others may discount his views or conclusions. To counteract this, he may bias his position even more (so-called "proactive exaggeration"). A survey of 300 readers of the British Medical Journal left no doubts — data from a "pain study" were considered to be of less interest, importance, relevance, validity and believability when the authors were thought to be employees of a fictitious drug company compared to a medical clinic.[5]

Do financial ties influence results reporting?

Review articles on the risk of passive smoking have come to very divergent conclusions. Barnes and Bero[2] analyzed 106 such review articles and observed that in 39 (37%), the authors did not report any health problems. Almost three quarters of these articles were written by persons with very close ties to the tobacco industry. Not surprisingly, the only statistically significant predictor of reporting no harm linked to passive smoking was investigator affiliation with the industry.

Stelfox et al.[10] reported the same year on a survey of authors who had published articles on the cardiovascular safety of calcium channel blockers. They

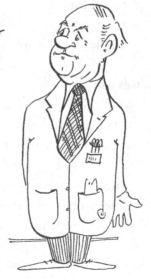

— A MOTHER IS A PERFECT
EXPERT ON HER CHILD,
BUT MAY NOT BE THE
MOST OBJECTIVE.

classified the articles as positive, neutral or critical. The authors of the articles were asked about their relationships with manufacturers of these drugs. For positive, neutral and critical articles, the proportion of authors with financial ties to industry was 96%, 60% and 37%, respectively. The authors concluded that the medical profession should develop stricter rules for avoiding financial conflicts of interest.

What is the evidence that industry trials produce more favorable results?

A large number of reports in leading medical journals have come to the same conclusion, namely, that sponsorship correlates with trial findings. One report[4] concluded that equipoise was maintained in studies funded by non-profit organizations — 53% of the trials favored the new product vs. 47% favoring standard treatment (p = 0.61). In contrast, 74% of industry sponsored studies favored the sponsor's new product while only 26% favored standard treatment (p = 0.004). Another study[7] reported that the authors' conclusions significantly and more often favored the new interventions if the trials were funded by for-profit organizations. In a systematic review of studies investigating the relationship between funding source and trial/meta-analysis outcomes, the authors[8] reported a summary odds ratio of 4.05 (95% CI 2.98-5.51). In other words, the likelihood of a favorable outcome was four times higher in trials sponsored by industry compared to trials sponsored by other sources.

When second-generation antipsychotics were tested against each other, 90% of 33 trials favored the sponsor's new drug.[6] The same two drugs were compared in nine of the 33 trials (five of which were sponsored by one company, and four by another). Eight of these nine studies reported results that favored the sponsor's drug. This is not a chance finding!

The most recent report[9] confirmed the previous observations. The proportion of trials favoring the sponsor's product was higher in drug trials funded by for-profit organizations (66% vs. 40% for non-profit organizations). The percentages were 82% vs. 50% for trials evaluating cardiovascular devices. It should come as no surprise that trials using surrogate outcomes were more likely to favor the sponsor than trials using clinical outcomes.

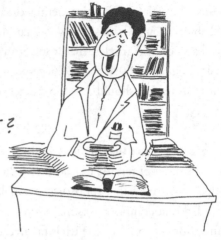

How are potential conflicts hidden?

Some authors with close ties to industry sometimes do not disclose their part-time affiliations with sponsors. Industry employees who maintain academic affiliations may also overlook their primary source of support. Silence about sponsorship, especially for major trials of new drugs, should raise a red flag. It goes without saying that many industry affiliated investigators and employees are highly independent and credible.

Key Points

- Be mindful of the great temptation to spin results to satisfy commercial sponsors.
- Industry sponsored trials are much more likely to report positive results compared to non-industry sponsored trials.
- Medical journals are trying to protect readers from misleading trial findings.

"Honesty is the best policy"

Chapter 21

Does publication in a reputable scientific journal guarantee quality?

Just because an article is published, even in a reputable medical journal, does not necessarily mean that it is scientifically credible. Several recent surveys[1,2,4] demonstrate that many journal publications not only fail to meet the highest methodological standards, but sometimes contain misleading conclusions. Readers must be prepared to evaluate scientific reports critically.

It is commonly assumed that articles published in peer-reviewed medical journals have passed stringent quality checks before publication. Most journals rely on referees with recognized expertise in a given field to scrutinize submitted manuscripts. This review, however, by no means assures quality in all instances. Although journal reviewers try to be thorough and fair in their evaluations, time constraints and other factors may lead to superficial reviews. Additionally, it is important to realize that this system of external peer review does not even exist for some scientific journals.

A former editor of the *New England Journal of Medicine*[6] describes journals' roles in assuring quality articles as follows — "In choosing manuscripts for

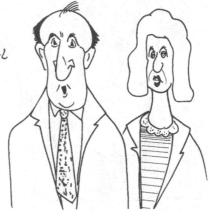

— WE JUST HAVE TO GET INTO
THE NEW ENGLAND JOURNAL
OR PEOPLE WON'T BELIEVE
OUR RESULTS.

publication, we make every effort to winnow out those that are clearly unsound, but we cannot promise that those we do publish are absolutely true... Good journals try to facilitate this process (of medical progress) by identifying noteworthy contributions from among the great mass of material that now overloads our scientific communication system. Everyone should understand, however, that this evaluative function is not quite the same thing as endorsement."

How representative are published articles?

The nature of a particular trial as well as the trial findings are likely to determine its destiny in the publication arena. Even the most prestigious medical journals depend on subscribers and advertisers. "Marketability" can serve as a powerful motivator to publish reports that not only address the latest scientific debates but also have fashionable overtones. It is also well known that trials reporting positive results (i.e., superior efficacy of the new or unproven treatment versus the standard or placebo treatment) have a much higher acceptance rate than negative findings in scientific journals. This so-called publication bias is a

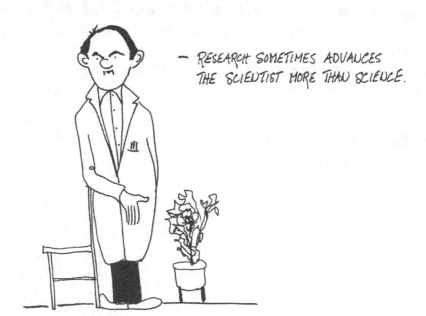

— RESEARCH SOMETIMES ADVANCES THE SCIENTIST MORE THAN SCIENCE.

concern.[7] It tends to give the readers a somewhat one-sided view of the evidence. For a fair assessment of a particular treatment, it is important to consider the totality of the trial evidence. Trials without favorable results may be just as important clinically as those with favorable findings. If a series of trials of the same intervention were conducted, the results would be distributed along a spectrum of outcomes. If those approaching one end of this spectrum receive "more press" through journal publication, the true treatment effect would not be known.

A group of investigators from the Swedish regulatory authority investigated 42 placebo-controlled trials of SSRIs.[3] Half of these had at least two publications; three trials contributed five publications each. Trials with significant effects were published more often as stand-alone reports. Many trials ignored the intention-to-treat analyses in favor of per- protocol analyses. Publication bias, as discussed in Chapter 5, is a major concern for investigators who conduct meta-analyses.

Is country of origin an issue?

There are two issues to consider — generalizability and quality. O'Shea and Califf[5] investigated intervention differences observed in large, international multicenter trials. They noted substantial variations among countries, in terms of patient characteristics, clinical procedures and observed event rates. In some of the trials, the country difference remained after adjustment for known risk factors. One would also expect differences in the level of patient care. Readers should be cautious about trial findings from countries with a system of patient care that is very different from their own. In reviewing results from multinational studies, attention should be paid to country or regional differences.

Vickers et al.[8] reviewed a large number of abstracts published between 1966 and 1995 and classified them based on treatment outcome. Three-quarters of the trial abstracts from the U.K. reported that the active treatments were better than the controls. This figure is not too surprising, considering the likelihood of publication bias. However, the corresponding percentages for China, the Soviet Union, Taiwan and Japan were 99, 97, 95 and 89%, respectively. No trials conducted in China and the Soviet Union reported that the study medication was ineffective. There are many potential explanations for these findings, publication bias being one of them. Questions about the quality and accuracy of the information have been raised. The pharmaceutical industry's increased engagement in trials conducted in developing countries (with very different medical systems, and limited research experience among the investigators) may not be in the best interest of medicine in high-income countries.

Key Points
- ⚬━ Publication of an article in a medical journal is not a guarantee of quality.
- ⚬━ The results of trials with negative findings often do not see the light of day (so-called publication bias).
- ⚬━ Caution is advised in accepting/extrapolating findings from countries with different health care systems.

"You can't tell a book by its cover"

Chapter 22

Is it necessary to be a biostatistician to interpret scientific data?

Many clinical trials employ statistical methods that are rarely taught in medical school or even in introductory biostatistics courses. It is easy to understand why a reader may be intimidated by the data analyses in clinical trial reports.

While collaboration with an experienced biostatistician is critical in designing, analyzing and interpreting a clinical trial, a good command of mathematics, clinical experience and common sense usually suffice for reviewing trial publications. Readers should be encouraged to form their own opinions, even if they consider their statistical knowledge to be limited. If you come across an article in which the authors report a p-value <0.05, but your judgment tells you that the treatment outcomes in the study groups are similar clinically, you probably have good reason to be skeptical. "Significant" in general parlance means meaningful. "Statistical significance" means that it is unlikely the differences are due to chance. Yet a statistically significant difference may not always be clinically meaningful. Likewise, an observed treatment group difference may be clinically important, yet fail to reach statistical significance.

Observed outcomes, such as means or proportions are called *point estimates*. Even if they do not reach statistical significance, differences in point estimates represent estimates of treatment effects. The lack of statistical significance means that observed differences between the treatment groups may have arisen by chance. Statistical tests may not be necessary in a few special cases, when the clinical course is unequivocal. For example, if three patients with advanced pancreatic cancer were cured by a new compound, this would be a truly remarkable clinical breakthrough, even though the numbers may be too small to reach statistical significance. As a rule, make a clinical judgment of the trial findings and do not rely solely on the reported or "promoted" p-value.

What is the role of trial size?

The size of a clinical trial should be considered when reviewing the results. Very large trials may report significant p-values associated with small treatment differences. P-values depend, in part, on the size of the trial. Moreover, if it takes 1,000 patients to demonstrate a statistically significant difference between two treatment approaches, one needs to put this finding in the proper clinical perspective. For the outcome of death or a serious morbid event with a favorable benefit to harm ratio, even very small differences may be clinically significant. If the outcome is of minor relevance to the patient, a statistically significant finding should not be overinterpreted. It is important to be sensitive to the distinctions between clinical and statistical significance, as well as to the importance of various outcomes.

Sample size is one of several factors that influences "statistical power" or "study power," defined as the ability to detect pre-specified intervention effects. The actual size of a mortality/morbidity clinical trial depends more on the number of observed events than on the number of enrolled participants. Trials

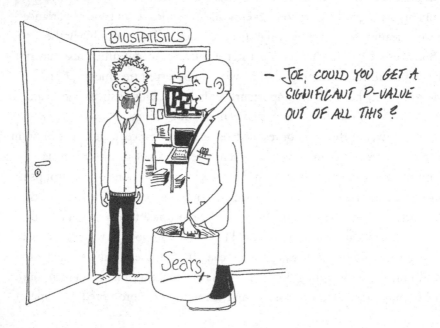

investigating a rare event or complication will require a very large population to accumulate enough events for proper testing. If the prophylactic effect of two antibiotics on the risk of deep wound infection is compared in 2,000 patients undergoing hip replacement surgery and the total number of treatment complications is 15, a statistically significant treatment group difference is not very likely. While a split by treatment group of 10 versus 5 may signal a 50% relative difference, it is not statistically significant. Since the difference can also be explained by chance, one would not want to base treatment recommendations on such numbers, even though the clinical importance associated with complications may be substantial. To make a claim of benefit, the best avenue would be to conduct a new and larger trial.

Clinical trials with small sizes or event rates may fail to demonstrate clinically significant results due to lack of statistical power. Even treatment effects as large as 20-30% that could have major clinical or public health significance, may be missed. Underpowered trials are commonplace in medicine. One solution to this problem is the pooling of results from several trials, as discussed in Chapter 5.

How can chance findings be avoided?
Another problem with small trials is their susceptibility to the play of chance. The influence of random variation and innovative *post hoc* hypothesis testing are behind many so-called breakthroughs reported from small trials.

Significance testing implies testing a pre-specified hypothesis. It is not possible to show statistically that two interventions are exactly equivalent. One can, however, test if they differ with varying degrees of precision. The stated "null hypothesis" makes the presumed assumption that the two treatments are identical with respect to the outcomes being assessed. If so, the two treatment groups represent samples from populations with the same distribution of outcomes.

If the observed difference between interventions is so large that it would be unlikely to have occurred if the null hypothesis were indeed true, the null hypothesis is rejected and the difference is considered to be statistically significant. A p-value of < 0.05 means that the probability (" p") is less than 5% that this difference could have occurred if the null hypothesis were true. It is a convention to define a p-value < 0.05 as statistically significant, meaning that we are willing to accept being wrong one time out of 20 if the null hypothesis is actually true.

Multiple statistical testing is another potential problem. There are two types: *repeated testing* of the same hypothesis during the course of a clinical trial (for example, as part of data monitoring) and *multiple testing* of different hypotheses. The major problem here is that every additional hypothesis tested increases the likelihood of rejecting the null hypothesis and declaring a difference to be statistically significant when, in fact, it may be due to chance. For example, if 10 true null hypotheses (i.e., no true differences) were to be tested in the same trial, there is a 40% probability of getting at least one p-value of <0.05.

It is difficult, and often unrealistic, to perform only one or two statistical tests as part of the final analyses. Several outcomes may be used to assess treatment benefit. Measurements may be obtained at various time points in a trial, and some measures (for example, the various domains of health-related quality of life) simply cannot be expressed as a single value. The proper way of dealing with repeated or multiple testing is to establish stricter criteria for declaring statistical significance. One approach is to require p-values to be much lower than 0.05 before considering them to be statistically significant (for example, dividing 0.05 by the number of tests being performed). According to

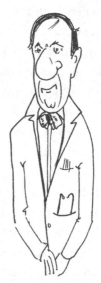

— SOMETIMES I HAVE TO GO THROUGH MANY DIFFERENT STATISTICIANS TO GET THE RIGHT RESULTS.

this conservative approach, if 10 tests are to be performed, each test's p-value would not be statistically significant unless it fell below 0.005. The advantage of this more stringent approach is that chance findings would not be declared statistically significant more often than 5 out of 100 times. The disadvantage is the increased risk of missing a true treatment effect. As a rule of thumb, the significance level (the p-value) should be adjusted when more than one significance test is conducted.

What's the danger with subgroup analyses?

It is common practice, at least in large-scale trials, to conduct subgroup analyses to determine treatment effect differences for various subsets of the entire study population. They are very common in trials that do not demonstrate an overall favorable trend. Such *post-hoc* explorations of the data are sometimes employed to find one or more subgroups in which the treatment "really works." What is often ignored is the mathematical fact that in any real or constructed data set with a trend in either direction, it is easy to single out at least one subgroup for which the difference reaches a conventional level of statistical significance.[3] The medical literature is replete with unconfirmed subgroup findings. Such *post-hoc* results should not be interpreted as conclusive. They may, however, be of value for hypothesis generation.

As an example of *post-hoc* analyses, take the case of a placebo-controlled trial of a calcium channel blocker in patients with acute myocardial infarction.[2] Although no overall mortality benefit from the active intervention was observed, a positive "trend" in the findings persuaded the investigators to perform subgroup analyses, which showed a significant reduction in mortality for infarction patients with normal myocardial function. The publication failed to report that mortality correspondingly increased in patients with impaired myocardial function, suggesting a negative inotropic drug effect. Additionally, this analytic exercise was not defined *a priori*. It should not be surprising that this *post-hoc* finding has yet to be confirmed in another calcium channel blocker trial.

The ISIS-2 trial tested the effects of streptokinase and aspirin, individually and in combination, on short-term mortality in patients admitted with acute myocardial infarction. The trial demonstrated mortality benefits for both active interventions. In a study of the potential fallacy of subgroup analyses, the investigators observed that patients born under the Zodiac signs of Gemini and Libra exhibited a 5% higher mortality on aspirin compared to placebo, whereas those born under the other Zodiac signs had a 30% lower mortality on aspirin compared to placebo.[1] There is no plausible biological explanation for this observation, which nicely illustrates the pitfalls of *post-hoc* subgroup analysis.

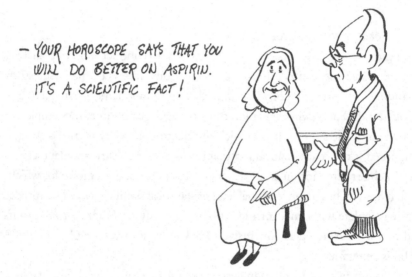

What is a confidence interval?

A perceived limitation of statistical significance testing is that the calculated p-value does not provide direct information about the magnitude of the effect size between two treatment approaches. For this reason, many investigators and medical journals favor a shift toward the use of *relative risk* (RR) and 95% *confidence intervals* (CI). The intervals put into perspective both the treatment effect and the probability of the observed difference. For example, a 95% CI provides information about the upper and lower boundaries of the observed treatment difference. The intervals would include the true treatment difference 95 times if tested 100 times. When the observed RR is not statistically significant, the 95% CI includes one, referred to as unity.

Assume that a long-term beta-blocker trial in survivors of acute myocardial infarction shows a 25% reduction in all-cause mortality with a 95% CI of 12-38%. A clinician may want to know the confidence that he or she can place on the observed 25% mortality reduction. The confidence interval tells him or her that a true benefit ranging from 12 to 38% is highly likely.

Key Points

- Statistical significance is not the same as clinical relevance.
- Treatment effects can be missed if trials are too small (i.e., underpowered).
- Multiple statistical testing requires adjustment of the p-value.
- Beware of *post-hoc* subgroup analyses.
- Confidence intervals provide valuable information for clinicians.

"There is safety in numbers"

Chapter 23

Are all drugs of a class interchangeable?

How are prescription drugs classified?

There are nearly 10,000 FDA-approved drugs available in the U.S. Grouping them together into various therapeutic classes, or by mechanism of action, makes sense in many respects. It helps clinicians remember the clinical indications for various drugs and how they work. Grouping also facilitates teaching, structures the regulatory approval process, and is the concernstone of drug development. Industry develops drugs representing new classes as well as additional members of established classes, so-called "me-too" drugs.

Although drug classification serves many purposes, it is far from perfect. It is based on the evidence that a group of drugs shares a single mechanism of action, such as blocking a particular enzyme.[1] The limitation lies in the fact that all drugs have multiple actions, favorable and unfavorable. Drugs within the same class have varying effects that are not necessarily associated with the class definition. These individual effects may be clinically very important and may explain essential differences between similar drugs of the same class. The belief that all drugs of a class are interchangeable is false.

What is the definition of a class effect?

Remarkably, there is no scientific definition for class effect.[2] Regulatory agencies have no definition either. The U.S. FDA uses a related term, class labeling, which is defined as follows: "All products within a class are assumed to be closely related in chemical structure, pharmacology, therapeutic activity, and adverse reactions." The qualifying term "assumed to be closely related" is not defined.

The pharmaceutical industry relies heavily on the class effect concept in promoting their "me-too" products. When several drugs of a class pass regulatory review and are approved for marketing, subsequent drugs of the same class appear to undergo less regulatory scrutiny. The promotion of these "me-too" drugs often takes advantage of the more extensive efficacy and safety documentation of their previously approved counterparts. Industry is willing to endorse the class concept when other drugs of a particular class have beneficial effects, but is less enthusiastic when one drug of a class is linked to harm.

Experience over the past decades has shown that drugs of the same class often differ in efficacy and safety. Since these differences cannot be predicted, the class effect concept and the notion that drugs are interchangeable should be viewed with caution. Two major determinants to consider relate to health efficacy and safety; many people include cost as a third factor.

What determines interchangeability for efficacy?

Similar effects on a surrogate marker represents a very unreliable indicator that one drug may be safely substituted for another. The limitations of these markers are discussed in Chapter 19. The fact that all ACE inhibitors lower elevated systolic blood pressure does not mean that all ACE inhibitors are interchangeable. Antihypertensive treatment is most meaningful when it is documented to have actual health benefits, i.e., reduction in risk of fatal and non-fatal stroke, myocardial infarction and heart failure.

A critical determinant of efficacy is drug dose. When determining whether or not drugs within a particular class are interchangeable, knowledge about equipotent dosing is important, but is all too often lacking. The approved or recommended doses of a drug are sometimes suboptimal. Quinopril in the recommended daily dose of 20 mg has no documented effect on ischemic events in patients after percutaneous coronary intervention.[5] Perindopril in the recommended daily dose of 4 mg had a moderate effect on blood pressure lowering, but did not reduce the risk of cardiovascular events in a large stroke prevention trial.[4] A strong dose-response relationship was demonstrated for enalapril in a study of 90-day rehospitalizations in patients with heart failure.[3] The higher the dose the lower the rate of rehospitalizations.

These examples illustrate the importance of drug dose. Any decision about interchangeability ought to take into account dose levels. The pertinent question should be "Which dose of new drug B is interchangeable with the proven optimal dose of approved drug A? A reliable answer can come only from a head-to-head mortality/morbidity trial comparing drugs A and B. It could be argued that

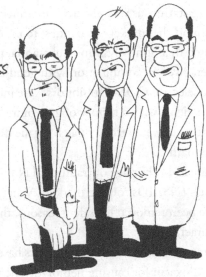

— ALL STATINS ARE ALIKE,
BUT OURS IS IN A CLASS
BY ITSELF.

outcome trials are necessary for all indications, but this is impractical. However, we believe that if an approved drug already exists for a specific indication and has proven benefit in terms of outcomes, any new drug in the class should be compared in at least one head-to-head trial to document equivalent benefit and the equi-effective dose.

What determines interchangeability for safety?

Even if drugs of the same class do have similar efficacy, they may differ in terms of their safety. Many examples illustrate this:

✔ Practolol, one of the first marketed beta-blockers, was shown to improve survival in post-infarction patients but was subsequently taken off the market for safety reasons.

✔ The late introduced calcium channel blocker, mibefradil, was approved for treatment of hypertension, but was later removed from the market due to adverse effects linked to drug-drug interactions.

✔ Troglitazone, the first marketed glitazone for treatment of Type 2 diabetes, was taken off the market due to liver toxicity, but was "replaced by" rosi- and pioglitazone.

✔   Cerivastatin was very effective in reducing LDL cholesterol, but it was taken off the market. In contrast to the other marketed statins, cerivastatin caused rhabdomyolysis in a substantial proportion of patients, especially when given in combination with gemfibrozil.

✔   The selective COX-2 inhibitors were introduced for pain relief, especially for patients with a history of gastrointestinal symptoms. Rofecoxib and valdecoxib were recently taken off the market, while celecoxib was allowed to remain.

✔   There is no shortage of traditional Non-Steroidal Anti-Inflammatory Drugs (NSAIDs) on the market. What is not well known is that five have been removed for safety reasons, the latest one being bromfenac (Duract).

✔   Two approved quinolone antibiotics have been removed from the market, temafloxacin for causing hemolytic anemia and grepafloxazin for causing QT-prolongation and increased risk of ventricular arrhythmias. A third, trovafloxazin (Trovan), had its use restricted for causing liver problems.

The list is much longer. Many drug classes have at least one harmful compound, which either did not make it to the market or was withdrawn due to major safety problems detected post-approval. Yet these harmful drugs were all as clinically effective as other members of their respective drug classes that remained on the market. Clearly, similar efficacy does not guarantee a similar safety profile.

How is interchangeability determined?

The answer is simple — in fair head-to-head comparisons. If the treatment outcome is a clinical event, the new trial should be designed to compare the two drugs, using this event as the primary outcome. Long-term safety should be determined in fair, long-term head-to-head comparisons.

"Me-too" drugs often rest their performance laurels on their approved "parent" predecessors. In our view, however, an untested drug ought to be considered an unproven drug. If given the choice between a proven early member of a drug class and a new, heavily promoted "me-too" version, go with the older, established drug.[2]

Key Points

- The class effect concept has no scientific definition.
- Many drug classes have at least one member pulled from development or marketing due to safety reasons.
- Similar efficacy is no guarantee of similar safety.
- Drugs of the same class should not be considered interchangeable without proof.

"Success has many fathers, but failure is an orphan"

Chapter 24

How much confidence can be placed on economic analysis?

What is the purpose of these analyses?

Several factors have contributed to the increasing attention focused on pharmaco-economic analyses. Society's desire to contain health care costs has put the pharmaceutical and device industries "on the defensive." Health care providers and regulatory agencies in a few countries are increasingly interested in cost-effectiveness. It is no longer a matter of simply asking, "How does a new therapy compare to the standard treatment in terms of cost?" The question is now multifaceted: "Are higher immediate and long-term costs likely to be associated with the new treatment?" "Are additional treatment expenses offset by improved quality of life or reduced morbidity?" "Is the additional cost associated with a marginal increase in benefit acceptable?" "Does the new, more expensive therapy lead to lower direct health care costs, i.e., fewer outpatient visits or hospitalizations or reduced need for costly procedures or laboratory tests — or does it reduce indirect costs by lowering absenteeism or premature death?"

Most new treatments add to the immediate medical cost, but the added cost may be offset by reducing medium and long-term expenditure. However, demonstrating how an expensive, efficacious compound is more cost-effective than a cheaper, less effective agent can be a challenge. A longitudinal study of ulcer patients[7] revealed that the introduction of H_2-blocker therapy increased the drug cost for ulcer treatment six- to seven-fold. The positive tradeoff was a five-fold decrease in the total cost of care for ulcer patients (including medication) due to reductions in ulcer surgeries, hospitalizations and outpatient visits. More comprehensive treatment programs for patients with Type 2 diabetes, including a marked increase in drug utilization, resulted in substantial savings in the annual health care cost per patient.[2] Good, unbiased comparisons of this type are needed so payers of healthcare and patients know what they are buying and for how much.

How reliable are cost-effectiveness studies?

In the absence of sound methodological standards, many cost-effectiveness studies, to date, have been of questionable quality. The most reliable studies are based on comprehensive patient databases from third party payers, health care providers, or national or state health departments. In contrast to clinical trials, these reflect very large, unselected patient populations, with cost figures that are derived from actual bills rather than projected or estimated bills. The overall costs of patient care are most meaningful if obtained from regional or managed-care databases that reflect hospitalizations, sick leave, outpatient visits and filled prescriptions.

Unfortunately, a large number of cost analyses are initiated by industry sponsors, which hire health economists who set out to demonstrate the specific advantages of a drug. Not surprisingly, most of these industry sponsored analyses favor the sponsors' product. In a systematic review of 494 studies, quality adjusted life years (QALY) were employed to compare the cost effectiveness of a broad spectrum of interventions.[1] The reported incremental cost effectiveness ratios were often below $20,000/QALY. Low ratios were 2 to 3 times more common in industry sponsored studies. In contrast, higher ratios were more common in studies with more rigorous methodology, or in those conducted in Europe and the U.S.

In a review of new drugs in oncology, it was found that trials funded by non-profit organizations were 8 times more likely to reach unfavorable cost-effectiveness conclusions (5 vs. 38%) compared with trials funded by pharmaceutical companies.[3] In contrast, favorable qualitative economic conclusions were 1.4 times more common in industry sponsored trials.

For drug approval and marketing of new drugs in Australia, pharmaco-economic analyses must indicate cost-effectiveness in some patient groups. An evaluation of 326 submissions between 1994-1997 revealed that 218 (67%) had "serious problems of interpretation."[4]

The potential for sponsorship bias was highlighted in a Sounding Board article in the New England Journal of Medicine[5] that called for disclosure of the financial arrangements between authors of cost-effectiveness articles and the manufacturers of the products studied. Shortly thereafter, the journal decided to restrict publication of cost effectiveness analyses funded by industry if any of the authors disclosed having direct ties with the sponsoring company.[6]

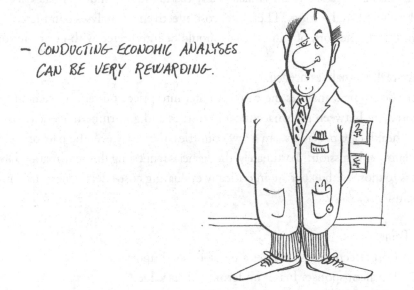

— CONDUCTING ECONOMIC ANALYSES CAN BE VERY REWARDING.

How useful are clinical trials for cost-effectiveness analysis?

Post hoc analyses of data derived from clinical trials designed to answer other research questions are perhaps the least reliable. Even if investigators pre-specify their intent to collect and analyze pharmaco-economic data, it is difficult to know the extent to which the hypotheses were pre-specified or whether the study is part of a *post-hoc* promotional campaign.

Even if sponsor bias could be eliminated, there is still the issue of whether or not the randomized clinical trial is the optimal vehicle for a cost-effectiveness study. The best cost data probably come from observational studies of actual clinical practice. Although it is convenient and efficient to collect additional cost data in a trial, this approach has its limitations. Enrolled patients represent a very highly selected group, which usually consists of younger low-risk individuals who are more likely to be free of co-morbid conditions. Trial-related clinic visits and laboratory procedures that are pre-specified in the study protocol do not necessarily reflect common practice patterns and their corresponding costs in primary care. In addition, the special attention given to trial participants may lead to early detection of problems directly or indirectly related to the study interventions. These and other factors can lead to over- or underestimates of cost in the clinical trial setting. Therefore, cost-effectiveness analyses conducted within the framework of clinical trials should be interpreted with great caution.

Why are these analyses needed?

Cost-effectiveness analyses increasingly enter into price and reimbursement negotiations between pharmaceutical industries and government agencies or other health care providers. In a few countries, they may even be part of a regulatory submission. Fortunately, the agencies requesting this information have access to those with expertise in critically evaluating cost-effectiveness data and conclusions.

Key Points

- ⌐ Cost effectiveness analyses are potentially important.
- ⌐ Prevalent sponsor biases undermine their value.
- ⌐ Clinical trials are unsuitable vehicles for cost-effectiveness analyses.

"A golden key can open any door"

Chapter 25

How should I handle the massive flow of information?

How massive is the flow?

It has been estimated that there are currently about 20,000 medical journals, with several hundred more being added each year. If we assume that each journal publishes 100 articles, that comes to around two million each and every year, and this number is growing exponentially. Needless to say, keep up with just a fraction of these, is a challenge. Fortunately, the situation is not as overwhelming as the numbers might suggest. Most of what is written is highly specialized and of limited relevance for clinical practice. For example, it's been estimated that less than 1% of oncology articles are important for practicing clinicians.[1]

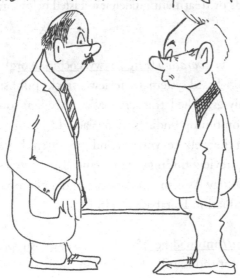

— HOW DO YOU KEEP UP WITH THE MEDICAL NEWS?
— ABC NEWS AND THE WALL STREET JOURNAL.

What is a reasonable survival strategy?

We recommend that you establish a search strategy that, without too much effort and time, will help to identify information relevant to you and your practice. If you are looking for a specific article, you should have no problems finding it on PubMed (www.pubmed.gov), which is available at no cost. To facilitate your search, enter one or more search terms, such as topic, authors or journal. You may also set limits to search within a specified time period, (i.e., 1999 to 2006). If a study was recently reported at a medical congress (and not yet published), you may find the news on www.pslgroup.com. Information about ongoing projects can be found on the many clinical trial registries, as discussed in Chapter 8.

If you are faced with a specific patient problem, are preparing for a lecture or want to know more about a therapy or the etiology or prognosis of a condition, there are many available medical literature databases. These can provide a list of relevant articles and sometimes even systematic reviews, which synthesize the information. Although, there is no one perfect resource for evidence-based medicine, clinicians can refer to many websites to find evidence-based answers to clinical questions. These include summarized, critically appraised resources prepared by experts, filtering tools that search for relevant content from a variety of resources and databases designed to retrieve relevant clinical trials or treatment guidelines. Listed below are several of these databases.

The Cochrane Collaboration (http://www.cochrane.org), which paved the way for evidence-based systematic reviews, tracks published clinical trials and meta-analyses. The latter serves as an excellent source for clinical evidence by combining findings from trials addressing the same scientific question. On the website, you can find specific study protocols and their corresponding review findings. Cochrane also provides access to a Health Technology Assessment database and a National Health Service Economic Evaluation Database (NHS EED).

PubMed (http://pubmed.gov) is a U.S. taxpayer-supported, web-based search engine for thousands of medical journals encompassing over 15 million indexed citations. PubMed offers two evidence-based databases to filter and narrow your search results: *Clinical Study Categories*, which identifies high quality studies limited to specific categories of interest and *Systematic Reviews*, which filters your results to include only systematic reviews.

FirstConsult (**http://firstconsult.com**) is a continually updated clinical information resource offering differential diagnosis, procedures, and 20,000 medical topics containing evidence-based summaries written by practicing physicians. Appropriate guidelines are included in the medical topics.

InfoPOEMs (**http://www.infopoems.com**) provides critically appraised articles by medical professionals that summarize and analyze important studies in major medical journals. Use the email alert service and receive new POEMs automatically.

InfoRetriever (**http://www.infopoems.com**) allows users to enter a topic and retrieve evidence-based information from medical texts, practice guidelines, the Cochrane Collaboration, critically appraised journal articles, "number needed to treat" data by disease/condition, clinical rules and calculators, images, internet resources, and patient education materials.

National Guidelines Clearinghouse (**http://guidelines.gov**) is a U.S. taxpayer-supported database of practice guidelines which allows the user to browse by disease, treatment, originating organization, or guidelines. A detailed search engine retrieves evidence-based guidelines by author, diagnosis, therapy, prevention, target population, or date of publication. Guidelines can be viewed side by side to compare recommendations from different sources.

Natural Medicines Comprehensive Database (**http://www.naturaldatabase.com**) is an ideal resource for answering patient questions about the effectiveness and safety of natural products and supplements. The database provides up-to-date, evidence-based clinical data on natural medicines, herbal medicines, and dietary supplements used in the western world and is compiled by pharmacists and physicians who are part of the *Pharmacist's Letter* and *Prescriber's Letter* research and editorial staff.

Health Web Evidence Based Healthcare (**http://healthweb.org**) is a website which links to many additional relevant resources. Readers could also consult their professional societies or an evidence-based medicine group within the society, a Medical Librarian or the National Network of Libraries of Medicine (1-800-338-7657) to find a local medical resource library and knowledgeable librarian.

What is your role in the critical appraisal of the literature?

When new articles appear that have a direct bearing on your field of work, you may wish to critically review them to determine whether the findings are relevant to your practice. There is an advantage in reviewing articles firsthand, rather than having them filtered through others who may have ties to the product being considered. Moreover, this approach also avoids the lag time between publication of original articles and their appearance in overview articles. Timely information is important since the half-life for "what's new in medicine" is short.

How would I go about it?

Most readers start off by reading the abstract. This usually provides a good summary and allows you to form a general opinion about the article. The introduction of the structured abstract markedly improved the quality of abstracts in general. In many cases, reviewing the abstract is all that is needed to determine whether the patient population, the intervention or the findings are of interest to you. If the abstract is relevant, read the full article to confirm the methods, findings and conclusions.

When reviewing the full article, you may wish to ask the questions noted in the following Table, many of which are part of a "checklist" from McMaster.[2,3] The optimal answer to questions 1 through 13 is "Yes,"as discussed in Appendix B. Each "No" or "Don't know" answer reflects a potential concern, with the level of concern increasing with each such answer.

Checklist for Critiquing a Clinical Trial Report*

Design

1.   Were patients randomized?
2.   Were patients unaware of treatment allocation?
3.   Were clinicians, and those collecting and adjudicating outcome data unaware of treatment allocation?
4.   Was the best alternative treatment administered as a comparator?
5.   Was the primary outcome both clearly specified and accurately measured?

Results

6.   Were the study groups similar with respect to known prognostic factors at baseline?
7.   Were nearly all patients treated and followed to study termination?
8.   Were patients analyzed in the group to which they were randomized?
9.   Was the result for the primary outcome clearly stated in the conclusion and supported by the confidence interval?
10. Were the adverse treatment effects adequately assessed?

Interpretation

11. Were the investigators free of potential conflicts-of-interest?
12. Was the sponsor an organization without vested interest in the outcome?
13. Were study limitations discussed?

Clinical Importance

14. Were the study patients similar to the patients in my practice?
15. Is the treatment benefit large enough to be important to my patients?

*The optimal answer to questions 1 through 13 is "Yes" (see Appendix B). Each "No" or "Don't know" answer reflects a potential concern, with the level of concern increasing with each such answer.

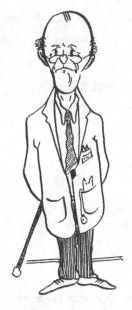

— I'M INSTINCTIVELY CRITICAL OF ALL
   PAPERS I HAVEN'T WRITTEN MYSELF.

Key points

- Familiarity with the medical literature is a strength.
- Available databases are a goldmine of information.
- First-hand knowledge is an antidote to one-sided information.
- A checklist can facilitate a critical appraisal.

"You can have too much of a good thing"

(Cato)

Chapter 26

How well is research translated into clinical care?

Annually, more than 10,000 clinical trials report their findings, thereby providing valuable opportunities for improved patient care. The challenge for health professionals is to translate this new knowledge into practice. A recent quality of care survey concluded that only 30-40% of patients in the Netherlands and in the United States were receiving optimal care.[4] The situation appears to be even more bleak when considering that 20-25% of the care administered was judged to be unnecessary or potentially harmful. A large U.S. study involving 30 acute or chronic conditions concluded that only 55% of patients received recommended care.[7] The most common deviation was undertreatment, which suggests that our national healthcare system as it exists today is failing us.

What is optimal care?

For a large number of medical conditions, evidence-based treatment guidelines (both national and international) have evolved through consensus among experts. Such guidelines, if unbiased, provide a strong basis for optimal care. The scientific evidence that forms the foundation for guidelines comes from high quality randomized clinical trials. The best treatment guidelines are updated on a regular basis to reflect new trial evidence. Even these, however, may involve subjective opinions. For example, findings from a clinical trial may be extrapolated to a broader patient group. Every extrapolation reflects a leap of faith, although the size of the leap may vary. If the upper age cutoff for enrollment into a trial was 70 years of age, it is highly likely that the trial results apply to 71 year old patients with the study condition. On the other hand, findings related to one particular drug and dose may not apply to other drugs, even within the same drug class. Other considerations that could invalidate extrapolations include concomitant conditions and co-interventions, which may alter treatment responses.

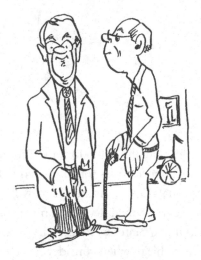

— TOO BAD THAT YOU ARE 71.
THERE IS AN EXCELLENT
TREATMENT FOR PEOPLE
UP TO 70 !

Do individual trials actually change practice?

Although the publication of a clinical trial with clear favorable or unfavorable results may not itself immediately change clinical practice, there are reports in the literature that describe striking temporal associations between publications of trials and changes in drug utilization.

Findings from the Coronary Drug Project indicated that the lipid-lowering agents clofibrate and niacin had no beneficial effect on mortality in survivors of myocardial infarction. During the years following the 1975 publication of these results, the number of patient visits involving prescription of lipid-lowering drugs dropped by more than half.[2] Interestingly, a 3-fold increase in such visits was observed almost a decade later following a publication reporting that cholestyramine reduced the incidence of fatal and non-fatal coronary heart disease.[2]

A survey of British physicians showed that the self-reported routine use of antiplatelet therapy (aspirin) rose from 9% to 84% within two years following publication of the Second International Study of Infarct Survival, which reported a substantial benefit of aspirin.[1] The use of aspirin after myocardial infarction also correspondingly increased over a three-year period in the U.S. (from 39 to 72%).[6] The authors additionally reported a decline in use of calcium antagonists post-infarction, after publication of a negative trial (from 57 to 33%).

The response to clinical trials is not, however, always so rapid. In a survey of physicians' attitudes towards two antiarrhythmic agents that had been shown in a landmark clinical trial to increase the risk of sudden death and all-cause mortality (encainide and flecainide),[8] 21% of surveyed physicians had not changed their use of these harmful agents and only 9% had stopped using them. Encainide was subsequently removed from the market.

What are the barriers to optimal care?
The barriers are many and exist at every stage of patient care.

Physicians play a major role in treatment decisions. They may disagree with treatment guidelines or they may be unwilling to follow what may be perceived as instructions on how to treat their patients. Many are influenced by industry's skillful marketing or other biases. Physicians may also lack critical appraisal skills and relevant knowledge.

Patients who stand to benefit the most from optimal care often have preconceived notions about their own care. More than one-third of adult Americans use "natural" or "alternative" products for health reasons, even though very limited evidence exists regarding their efficacy and safety. Adherence to prescribed long-term therapies may be poor, due to patients receiving incomplete information about the therapeutic benefits of the medicines they take. Other patients may avoid taking proven therapies, due to fears of rare adverse drug reactions.

Payers of health care and hospitals must address the escalating costs of patient care. Financial considerations may lead to certain restrictions, especially with regard to utilization of costly drugs or procedures. The emphasis of purchasing contracts is often on expense rather than effectiveness, and decisions are sometimes based on limited documentation.[5]

The *pharmaceutical industry* has a major influence on the quality of care. To a large extent it determines the design of the trials being conducted, whether they are reported, as well as when and where they are reported. Large budgets support the skillful marketing of a company's product, with little regard to its actual efficacy compared to other compounds. Many of these promotional strategies would not be effective if the medical profession were better informed and more critical.

The *regulatory agencies* play an important role in the approval of new products. Randomized clinical trials provide critical information regarding efficacy. The agencies could contribute to improving care if they improved safety monitoring post-approval and incorporated more evidence-based data on treatment alternatives in the drug labeling.

Politicians could improve the quality of care by becoming more involved in evaluating how the financial resources they provide are being spent and by requiring greater accountability. There is a substantial waste in medicine. Purchasing contracts that place more emphasis on cost savings than on scientific documentation are penny-wise but pound-foolish. Cheaper me-too drugs may be less effective and/or more harmful than the better documented original members of a drug class.

What are the solutions?

Many of the parties involved are now directing more attention to quality improvement. Recently introduced performance measures are a step in the right direction. Audits of performance measures followed by feedback, including rankings, are very effective in increasing awareness and improving care.[9] Clinicians and institutions seem to be more than willing to change behavior if they rank low compared to their counterparts. Unfortunately, most performance measures focus on processes (prescription of a specific medication or performance of a specific diagnostic test) rather than on clinical outcomes.[3] Financial incentives that reward the application of evidence-based practice have also been introduced.

You could also contribute by being a more critical consumer of medical information. A healthy dose of skepticism is needed to counterbalance the often incomplete and biased information being reported by those with ties to the product being promoted. Our hope is that this text has introduced you to critical appraisal and reminded you that all that glitters is not gold.

Key points

⚬ᴦ Every effort should be made to provide optimal or evidence-based medicine.

⚬ᴦ There are a large number of barriers to optimal care.

⚬ᴦ Patients expect to get the best possible care.

⚬ᴦ Efforts to stimulate better patient care are showing promise.

"What everybody says must be true"

A

active-control treatment A control treatment that involves use of a pharmacologically or medically active substance.

adherence The extent to which patients follow the prescribed treatment regimen. The terms "compliance" and "adherence" are often used interchangeably.

adverse drug reaction (ADR) Any undesirable effect of a drug beyond its anticipated therapeutic effects occurring during clinical use.

alternative hypothesis An alternative to the null hypothesis that specifies some true underlying difference between two or more populations or groups.

analysis by treatment administered Allows withdrawal from the analysis of participants who, for whatever reasons, have not adhered to the treatment protocol. Thus, the data are analyzed by treatment actually administered rather than by treatment assigned.

a priori Formed or conceived beforehand.

B

baseline assessment Assessment of subjects as they enter a trial and before they receive any treatment.

bias A preconceived personal preference or inclination that influences the way in which a measurement, analysis, assessment or procedure is performed or reported.

blinding/masking A procedure in which one or more parties to the trial are kept unaware of the treatment assignment(s). Single-blinding usually refers to the subject(s) being unaware, and double-blinding usually refers to the subject(s), investigator(s), monitor, and, in some cases, data analyst(s) being unaware of the treatment assignment(s).

C

comparator An investigational or marketed product (i.e., active-control), or placebo, used as a reference in a clinical trial.

compliance The extent to which patients follow the prescribed treatment regimen. The terms "compliance" and "adherence" are often used interchangeably.

composite event An event that is considered to have occurred if any one of several different outcomes are observed (e.g., occurrence of an attack of angina pectoris, a transient ischemic attack, or a myocardial infarction in a trial using a composite vascular event as the outcome measure).

confidence interval (CI) The confidence interval quantifies uncertainty. The 95% CI is the range of values within which we can be 95% sure that the true value lies for the whole population of patients from whom the study patients were selected. The CI narrows as the number of patients on which it is based increases.

continuous variable A variable that is capable of assuming any value over a specified range.

D

data dredging A term used to characterize analyses that are done on an *ad hoc* basis, without benefit of prestated hypotheses, as a means of identifying noteworthy differences.

Data Monitoring Committees (Data and Safety Monitoring Board) An independent data-monitoring committee that may be established by the sponsor to assess at intervals the progress of a clinical trial, the safety data, and the critical efficacy endpoints, and to recommend to the sponsor whether to continue, modify or stop a trial.

Declaration of Helsinki Recommendations about conducting biomedical research involving human subjects adopted by the 18th World Medical Assembly in Helsinki in 1974. (See reference #18 in Chapter 17).

dichotomous variable A discrete variable that has only two possible values. Binary variable.

double-blind study A study in which neither the subject nor the investigator knows what treatment a subject is receiving.

E

evidence-based medicine An approach to practice and teaching that integrates pathophysiological rationale, caregiver experience, and patient preferences with valid and current clinical research evidence.

exclusion criteria A list of criteria, any one of which excludes a potential subject from participation in a study.

F

FDA Food and Drug Administration (USA)

feasibility study A preliminary study designed to determine the practicality of a larger study.

G

Good Clinical Practice (GCP) A standard for the design, conduct, performance, monitoring, auditing, recording, analyses, and reporting of clinical trials that provides assurance that the data and reported results are credible and accurate, and that the rights, integrity, and confidentiality of trial subjects are protected.

H

Hawthorne effect A tendency for people to change their behavior because they are the targets of special interest and attention in a research study.

I

ICH International Conference on Harmonisation of Technical Requirements for Registration of Pharmaceuticals for Human Use

inclusion criteria The criteria that prospective subjects must meet to be eligible for participation in a study.

informed consent A process by which a subject voluntarily confirms his or her willingness to participate in a particular trial, after having been informed of all aspects of the trial that are relevant to the subject's decision to participate. Informed consent is documented by means of a written, signed and dated informed consent form.

Institutional Review Board (IRB) An independent body constituted of medical, scientific, and non-scientific members, whose responsibility it is to ensure the protection of the rights, safety and well-being of human subjects involved in a trial by, among other things, reviewing, approving, and providing continuing review of trial protocol and of the methods and material to be used in obtaining and documenting informed consent of the trial subjects.   Other names for such bodies include independent review board, independent ethics committee, committee for the protection of human subjects.

intention-to-treat analysis Requires that no randomized participants can be withdrawn from the analysis.

interim analysis Any data analysis carried out during the trial for the purpose of treatment effects monitoring.

investigator A person responsible for the conduct of the clinical trial at a trial site. If a trial is conducted by a team of individuals at a trial site, the investigator is the responsible leader of the team and may be called the principal investigator.

M

monitoring The act of overseeing the progress of a clinical trial, and of ensuring that it is conducted, recorded, and reported in accordance with the protocol,

Standard Operating Procedures (SOPs), Good Clinical Practice (GCP), and the applicable regulatory requirement(s).

multicenter trial A clinical trial conducted according to a single protocol but at more than one site, and therefore, carried out by more than one investigator.

multiple looks A term used to refer to the fact that treatment comparisons are made at various time points over the course of a trial.

multiple outcomes A term used to refer to the fact that a trial involves several different outcome measures, each of which is used or is to be used to make treatment comparisons.

N

null hypothesis A hypothesis that postulates no underlying difference in the populations or groups being compared with regard to the characteristic or condition of interest.

number needed to treat (NNT) The number of patients who need to be treated to achieve one additional favorable outcome.

O

off-label use Use of an approved drug outside the approved indication(s).

outcome variable An observation variable recorded for patients in the trial at one or more time points after enrollment for the purpose of assessing the effects of the study treatments.

P

phase I trial The first stage in testing a new drug in man. The studies are usually done to generate preliminary information on the chemical action and safety of the drug using normal healthy volunteers. Usually done without a comparison group.

phase II trial The second stage in testing a new drug in man. Generally carried out on patients with the disease or condition of interest. The main purpose is to provide preliminary information on treatment efficacy and to supplement information on safety obtained from phase I trials. Usually, but not always, designed to include a control treatment and random allocation of patients to treatment.

phase III trial The third stage in testing a new drug in man. Concerned primarily with assessment of dosage effects and efficacy and safety. Usually designed to include a control treatment and random allocation to treatment. Once this phase is completed the drug manufacturers may request permission to market the drug.

phase IV trial Generally, a randomized controlled trial that is designed to evaluate the long-term safety and efficacy of a drug for a given indication. Usually carried out after licensure of the drug for that indication.

pilot study A preliminary study designed to indicate whether a larger study is practical. See feasibility study.

placebo A pharmacologically inactive agent often given to controls in clinical trials

post hoc Formulated after the fact

postmarketing surveillance Ongoing safety monitoring of marketed drugs.

power The probability of rejecting the null hypothesis when it is false.

primary outcome variable The outcome variable that is designated or regarded as key in the design or analysis of the results of a trial. Generally, the variable used for sample size calculations in the design of the trial or, when no sample size calculation is made, for the main avenue of data analyses.

protocol A document that describes the objective(s), design, methodology, statistical considerations, and organization of a trial. The protocol usually also gives the background and rationale for the trial, but these could be provided in other protocol referenced documents.

publication bias Results from the fact that studies with positive results are more likely to be published.

p-value A value associated with an observed test statistic that indicates the probability that a value as extreme or more extreme than the one observed will arise by chance alone in repeated replications of the study.

Q

QoL quality of life

R

random allocation Assignment of subjects to treatment or control group in an unpredictable way. Assignment sequences are concealed, but available for disclosure in the event a subject has an adverse experience.

randomization The process of assigning trial subjects to treatment or control groups using an element of chance to determine the assignments in order to reduce bias.

recruitment Process that employs inclusion and exclusion criteria and is used by investigators to enroll appropriate subjects into a clinical study.

regression to the mean A phenomenon that occurs when a second determination or measurement is made on those individuals with an extreme initial determination or measurement. On average, the second determination or measurement tends to be less extreme than the initial one.

S

sample size calculation A mathematical calculation, usually carried out when a trial is planned, that indicates the number of patients to be enrolled in order to provide a specified degree of statistical precision for a specified type I and type II error protection.

serious adverse event (SAE) or serious adverse drug reaction (serious ADR) Any untoward medical occurrence that at any dose results in death, is life threatening, requires inpatient hospitalization or prolongation of existing hospitalization, results in persistent or significant disability/incapacity, or is a congenital anomaly/birth defect.

sponsor An individual, company, institution, or organization which takes responsibility for the initiation, management, and/or financing of a clinical trial.

stratified allocation A method of treatment assignment in which patients are first classified into defined subgroups based on one or more baseline variable and then assigned to treatment within the defined subgroups.

subgroup A subpart of the study population distinguished by a particular characteristic or set of characteristics (e.g., males under age 45 at entry).

surrogate outcome A laboratory measurement or a physical sign used as a substitute for a clinically meaningful endpoint that measures directly how a patient feels, functions or survives.

systematic review A review in which evidence on a topic has been systematically identified, appraised and summarized according to predetermined criteria.

T

type I error (statistics) The probability of rejecting the null hypothesis when it is true, usually denoted by the Greek letter α.

type II error (statistics) The probability of accepting the null hypothesis when it is false, usually denoted by the Greek letter β.

Design

1. **Were patients randomized?**
   Randomization is an essential design feature because it tends to produce study groups that are comparable with respect to known and unknown risk factors, removes investigator bias in the allocation of patients and guarantees that statistical tests will have valid significance levels. Non-randomized trials are especially susceptible to bias in favor of the new treatment.

   You can determine if a trial includes randomized groups from the Methods section of the journal article or in the Abstract. If a clinical trial report does not clearly state that participants were randomized to the active and control groups it is safe to assume that randomization was not used.

2. **Were patients unaware of treatment allocation?**
   Single-blind designs, whereby patients do not know which study drug they are receiving, reduce or avoid problems of biased patient reporting of symptoms and adverse effects. Patients, like clinicians, often have preconceived notions, hopes or expectations that the new treatment is better.

   The Methods section or the Abstract should specifically state whether the trial was "single-blind," (sometimes stated "participants were blinded to treatment assignment"). Participants are also blinded in a "double-blind" design.

3. **Were clinicians, and those collecting and adjudicating outcome data unaware of treatment allocation?**
   Double-blind designs, whereby investigators are also unaware of treatment assignment, minimize the potential problem of clinician/investigator bias during data collection and event adjudication. It reduces the possible influence of preconceived notions.

   The Methods section or the Abstract should specifically state whether the trial was "double-blind," (sometimes stated "both participants and study clinicians (or investigators) were blinded to treatment assignment"). Open-label studies are not blinded.

4. **Was the best alternative treatment administered as a comparator?**
    There is an ethical mandate requiring the comparator in any active-control trial to
    be the optimal available treatment. Patients should never be denied the current
    standard of care. New drugs can be tested against best treatments or in addition
    to best treatments. The use of a placebo is appropriate only when no standard
    treatment is available.

    If evidence is not provided in the trial report that the comparator was the optimal
    or preferred standard treatment, you must use your clinical judgment to
    determine whether that was the case.

5. **Was the primary outcome both clearly specified and accurately measured?**
    Pre-specification of the primary outcome, including its definition and ascertain-
    ment, is a fundamental requirement. Deviations open the door to bias and should
    reduce the confidence in the reported findings. If not clearly stated in the article,
    this information may be obtained from the trial protocol, which should be available
    through a web-based trial registry.

    A vague or general statement about the trial objective(s) at the end of the
    Introduction should raise concerns. This opens the door to post-hoc changes in
    the pre-specified primary outcome, which are sometimes done to fit the study
    results.

Results

6. **Were the study groups similar with respect to known prognostic
    factors at baseline?**
    Knowledge of baseline comparability for prognostic factors is important for the
    proper interpretation of trial results. Known and unknown imbalances can distort
    trial results.

    The report typically includes a Table showing the comparability of study groups.
    If, despite randomization, the groups are clearly imbalanced for major prognostic
    factors, the final analysis should take this into account.

7. **Were nearly all patients treated and followed to study termination?**
   Good adherence of patients to the prescribed treatment regimens for the duration of the trial is essential to answer the trial questions. High non-adherence rates should be a concern, since they are often treatment-related. Claims of treatment benefits in trials with high non-adherence should be interpreted with caution. High rates of missing data are a reflection of the overall quality of a trial. They are particularly alarming if they differ between the study groups.

   The adherence rates over time should be reported for each treatment group.

8. **Were patients analyzed in the group to which they were randomized?**
   The final analyses should be performed according to patients' original treatment group assignments, regardless of whether or not they followed the protocol as intended. This "intention-to-treat analysis" is the preferred analytic approach and should never be replaced by "per treatment administered analysis." Excluding randomized patients from the analysis undermines the benefits of randomization and can lead to biased results of unknown magnitude or direction.

   The Methods section should state whether the analysis used an intention-to-treat approach. Any deviation from this standard calls for exercising caution when interpreting the results.

9. **Was the result for the primary outcome clearly stated in the conclusion and supported by the confidence interval?**
   The major conclusion(s) of any clinical trial should be based on the findings of the pre-specified primary outcome. Because deviations from this fundamental principle are common, journal readers should be on their guard when reviewing trial results. Non-significant statistical findings for the primary outcome may be overinterpreted. Nominally statistically significant findings for one or more of several pre-specified secondary outcomes may be highlighted rather than drawing attention to a non-significant primary outcome.

   All reports should present 95% confidence intervals around the observed treatment results for the primary outcome. Wide confidence intervals including 1.0 and confidence intervals with lower or upper boundaries approaching 1.0, should be interpreted with caution.

10. **Were the adverse treatment effects adequately assessed?**
A full accounting of all adverse effects and events is crucial for determining the benefit-harm balance. If you sense that drug safety is not fully disclosed, worry about the trial findings.

The report should state which adverse effects were measured. Use your clinical judgment to decide if the reporting was adequate and complete. If not, be cautious of the result.

Interpretation

11. **Were the investigators free of potential conflicts-of-interest?**
Investigators with potential conflicts-of-interest (COI) are more likely to report favorable results and conclusions compared to investigators without COIs. Articles without disclosure statements may not rule out potential conflicts. These reports should be interpreted with the same caution reserved for those in which COI is disclosed.

Disclosures are typically found at the end of the Discussion section.

12. **Was the sponsor an organization without vested interest in the outcome?**
Trials with commercial sponsors are much more likely to report results that are favorable to the sponsor's products compared to trials with non-commercial sponsors. Trials comparing two active drugs overwhelmingly favor the sponsor's product.

The source of funding is also given at the end of the Discussion section.

13. **Were study limitations discussed?**
There is no perfect trial. The investigators know the limitations of their trials and ought to comment on them in their published reports. This provides readers with added insights and enhances the credibility of the study being reported.

The limitations of a trial are typically presented in the Discussion. Failure to discuss trial limitations is a weakness.

Clinical Importance

14. **Were the study patients similar to the patients in my practice?**
    Patients enrolled in clinical trials are typically at lower risk (younger, less co-morbidity and co-intervention) than patients in general practice. Therefore, the treatment benefits in your patients may be smaller and the adverse effects more common, especially in older patients with co-morbidities and co-interventions.

15. **Is the treatment benefit large enough to be important to my patients?**
    The question to ask is "Does the new treatment *add value* to treatments already available?" This could involve greater benefit, fewer adverse effects and/or lower cost. Since cost is typically higher for newer treatments, this consideration should be weighed against the other two factors.

References

About the Authors
1.   Friedman LM, Furberg CD, DeMets DL. *Fundamentals of Clinical Trials.* New York, Springer-Verlag, 1998 (3rd ed.).

2.   DeMets DL, Furberg CD, Friedman LM, eds. *Data Monitoring in Clinical Trials. A Case Studies Approach.* New York, Springer, 2006.

Chapter 1
1.   Friedman LM, Furberg CD, DeMets DL. *Fundamentals of Clinical Trials.* New York, Springer-Verlag, 1998 (3rd ed.).

2.   Piantadosi S. *Clinical Trials: A Methodologic Perspective.* New York, John Wiley & Sons, Inc., 1997.

3.   Pocock S. *Clinical Trials: A Practical Approach.* West Sussex, England, John Wiley & Sons, Ltd., 1983.

4.   Simpson J, Speake J. *The Concise Oxford Dictionary of Proverbs.* Oxford, Oxford University Press, 1998.

5.   Berra Y. *The Yogi Book. "I Really Didn't Say Everything I Said."* New York, Workman Publishing, 1998.

Chapter 2
1.   National Association of Attorneys General. Settlement: Fifty Attorney Generals announce settlement with Pfizer over improper off-label drug marketing. http://www.naag.org/issues/20040513-settlement-pfizer.php.

2.   Radley DC, Finkelstein SN, Stafford RS. Off-label prescribing among office-based physicians. *Arch Intern Med* 2006;166:1021-1026.

Chapter 3
1.   Friedman LM, Furberg CD, DeMets DL. *Fundamentals of Clinical Trials.* New York, Springer-Verlag, 1998 (3rd ed.).

2.   Guidance for Industry. E6 Good Clinical Practice: Consolidated Guidance. ICH, April 1996. www.fda.gov/cder/guidance/959fnl.pdf.

3.   Hypertension Detection and Follow-up Program Cooperative Group: Five-year findings of the Hypertension Detection and Follow-up Program. Reduction in mortality of persons with high blood pressure, including mild hypertension. *JAMA* 1979;242:2562-71.

4.   Karlowski TR, Chalmers TC, Frenkel LD, et al. Ascorbic acid for common cold. A prophylactic and therapeutic trial. *JAMA* 1975;231:1038-42.

5.   Parsons HM. What happened at Hawthorne? *Science* 1974;183:922-32.

6.   Vandenbroucke JP. Benefits and harms of drug treatments. *Br Med J* 2004;329:2-3.

Chapter 4
1.   Bailey DG, Malcolm J, Arnold O, et al. Grapefruit juice-drug interactions. 1998. *Br J Clin Pharmacol* 2001;52:216-7.

2.   Cleland JG, Cohen-Solal A, Aguilar JC, et al. Management of heart failure in primary care (the IMPROVEMENT of Heart Failure Programme): an international survey. *Lancet* 2002;360:1631-9.

3.   Connolly H, Crary JL, McGoon MD, et al. Valvular heart disease associated with fenfluramine-phentermine. *N Engl J Med* 1997;337:581-8.

4.   Källén BA, Otterblad-Olausson P, Danielsson B. Is erythromycin therapy teratogenic in
        humans? *Reprod Toxicol* 2005; 20:209-14.

5.   Kernan WN, Viscoli CM, Brass LM, et al. Phenylpropanolamine and the risk of hemorrhagic
        stroke. *N Engl J Med* 2000;343:1826-32.

6.   Laughren T. Premarketing studies in the drug approval process: understanding their limitations
        regarding the assessment of drug safety. *Clin Ther* 1998;20 Suppl C:C12-9.

7.   Mortimer Ö (1999). Personal communication.

8.   Venning GR. Identification of adverse reactions to new drugs II: how were 18 important
        adverse reactions discovered and with what delays? *Br Med J* 1983;286:289-92.

9.   World Medical Association Declaration of Helsinki. Ethical principles for medical research
        involving human subjects. *JAMA* 2000;284:3043-5.

Chapter 5
1.   Alderson P, Roberts I. Corticosteroids in acute traumatic brain injury: systematic review of
        randomised controlled trials. *Br Med J* 1997;314:1855-9.

2.   Cochrane Injuries Group Albumin Reviewers. Human albumin administration in critically ill
        patients: systematic review of randomised controlled trials. *Br Med J* 1998;317:235-40.

3.   CRASH Trial Collaborators. Effect of intravenous corticosteroids on death within 14 days in
        10008 adults with clinically significant head injury (MRC Crash trial): randomized placebo-
        controlled trial. *Lancet* 2004;364:1321-8.

4.   Jüni P, Nartey L, Reichenback S, Sterchi R, Dieppe PA, Egger M. Risk of cardiovascular
        events and rofecoxib: cumulative meta-analysis. *Lancet* 2004:364:2021-9.

5.   LeLorier J, Gregoire G, Benhaddad A, et al. Discrepancies between meta-analyses and
        subsequent large randomized, controlled trials. *N Engl J Med* 1997;337:536-42.

6.   Rothstein H, Sutton A, Borenstein M (eds). *Publication Bias in Meta-analysis: Prevention,
        Assessment, and Adjustments.* London, John Wiley & Sons, Ltd., 2005.

7.   The SAFE Study Investigators: A comparison of albumin and saline for fluid resuscitation in
        the intensive care unit. *N Engl J Med* 2004;350:2247-56.

8.   Sauerland S, Maegele M. A CRASH landing in severe head injury. *Lancet* 2004;364:1291-2.

9.   Young D. ASHP News: Congress investigates FDA's handling of antidepressant safety
        information. November 1, 2004. http://www.ashp.org/news/ShowArticle.cfm?id=8375.

Chapter 6
1.   Doll R, Hill AB. The mortality of doctors in relation to their smoking habits. A preliminary
        report. *Br Med J* 1954;4877:1451-5.

2.   Doll R, Peto R, Boreham J, et al. Mortality in relation to smoking: 50 years' observations on
        male British doctors. *Br Med J* 2004;328:1519-27.

3.   Kernan WN, Viscoli CM, Brass LM, et al. Phenylpropanolamine and the risk of hemorrhagic
        stroke. *N Engl J Med* 2000;343:1826-32.

4.   McBride WG. Thalidomide and congenital abnormalities. *Lancet* 1961;278:1358.

5.   Venning GR. Identification of adverse reactions to new drugs II: how were 18 important adverse reactions discovered and with what delays? *Br Med J* 1983;286:289-92.

Chapter 7
1.   Hulley S, Grady D, Bush T, et al., Randomized trial of estrogen plus progestin for secondary prevention of coronary heart disease in post-menopausal women. Heart and Estrogen/progestin Replacement Study (HERS) Research Group. *JAMA* 1998;280:605-13.

2.   Jick H, Zornberg GL, Jick SS, et al. Statins and the risk of dementia. *Lancet* 2000;356:1627-31.

3.   Petitti DB. Hormone replacement therapy and heart disease prevention. Experimentation trumps observation. *JAMA* 1998;280:650-2.

4.   Rockwood K, Kirkland S, Hogan DB, et al. Use of lipid-lowering agents, indication bias, and the risk of dementia in community-dwelling elderly people. *Arch Neurol* 2002;59:223-7.

5.   Venning GR. Validity of anecdotal reports of suspected adverse drug reactions: the problem of false alarms. *Br Med J* 1982;284:249-52.

6.   Wolozin B, Kellman W, Ruosseau P, et al. Decreased prevalence of Alzheimer disease associated with 3-hydroxy-3 methyglutaryl coenzyme A reductase inhibitors. *Arch Neurol* 2000;57:1439-43.

7.   Writing Group for the Women's Health Initiative Investigators. Risks and benefits of estrogen plus progestin in healthy postmenopausal women. Principal results from the Women's Health Initiative randomized controlled trial. *JAMA* 2002;288:321-33.

Chapter 8
1.   Chan A-W, Hróbjartsson A, Haahr MT, et al. Empirical evidence for selective reporting of outcomes in randomized trials. Comparison of protocols to published articles. *JAMA* 2004;291:2457-65.

2.   Chan A-W, Krleza-Jeric K, Schmid I, et al. Outcome reporting bias in randomized trials funded by the Canadian Institutes of Health Research. *CMAJ* 2004;171:735-40.

3.   DeAngelis CD, Drazen JM, Frizelle FA, et al. Clinical trial registration: a statement from the International Committee of Medical Journal Editors. *JAMA* 2004;292:1363-4.

4.   Goudie RB. The birthday fallacy and statistics of Icelandic diabetes. *Lancet* 1981;2:1173.

5.   Haug C, Gøtzsche PC, Schroeder TV. Registries and registration of clinical trials. *N Engl J Med* 2005;353:2811-2.

6.   Sears MR, Taylor DR, Print CG, et al. Regular inhaled β-agonist treatment in bronchial asthma. *Lancet* 1990;336:1391-6.

7.   Sim I, An-Wen C, Gülmezoglu AM, et al. Clinical trial registration: transparency is the watchword. *Lancet* 2006;367:1631-3.

8.   Zarin DA, Tse T, Ide NC. Trial registration at ClinicalTrials.gov between May and October 2005. *N Engl J Med* 2005;353:2779-87.

Chapter 9
1.   Hansson L, Lindholm LH, Niskanen L, et al. Effect of angiotensin-converting-enzyme inhibition compared with conventional therapy on cardiovascular morbidity and mortality in hypertension: the Captopril Prevention Project (CAPPP) randomised trial. *Lancet* 1999;353:611-6.

2.   Peto R. Failure of randomization by "sealed" envelope. *Lancet* 1999;354;73.

Chapter 10
1.   Hulley S, Grady D, Bush T, et al., Randomized trial of estrogen plus progestin for secondary
        prevention of coronary heart disease in post-menopausal women. Heart and Estrogen/
        progestin Replacement Study (HERS) Research Group. *JAMA* 1998;280:605-13.

2.   Karlowski TR, Chalmers TC, Frenkel LD, et al. Ascorbic acid for common cold. A prophylactic
        and therapeutic trial. *JAMA* 1975;231:1038-42.

Chapter 11
1.   DuBeau CE, Yalla SV, Resnick NM. Implications of the most bothersome prostatism symptom
        for clinical care and outcomes research. *J Amer Geriatr Soc* 1995;43:985-92.

Chapter 12
1.   Croog SH, Levine S, Testa MA et al. The effects of antihypertensive therapy on the quality of
        life. *N Engl J Med* 1986;314:1657-64.

2.   Jachuck SJ, Brierley H, Jachuck S, et al. The effect of hypotensive drugs on the quality of life.
        J R Coll Gen Pract 1982;32:103-5.

Chapter 13
1.   DeMets DL, Califf RM. Lessons learned from recent cardiovascular clinical trials: Part I.
        Circulation 2002;106:746-751.

2.   Echt DS, Liebson PR, Mitchell LB, et al. Mortality and morbidity in patients receiving
        encainide, flecanide or placebo. The Cardiac Arrhythmia Suppression Trial. *N Engl J Med*
        1991;324:781-8.

3.   Fleming TR, DeMets DL. Surrogate end points in clinical trials: Are we being mislead? *Ann
        Intern Med* 1996;125:605-13.

4.   Hulley S, Grady D, Bush T, et al., Randomized trial of estrogen plus progestin for secondary
        prevention of coronary heart disease in post-menopausal women. Heart and Estrogen/
        progestin Replacement Study (HERS) Research Group. *JAMA* 1998;280:605-13.

5.   Riggs BL, Hodgson SF, O'Fallon WM, et al. Effect of fluoride treatment on the fracture rate in
        postmenopausal women with osteoporosis. *N Engl J Med* 1990;322:802-9.

6.   Temple RJ. A regulatory authority's opinion about surrogate endpoints. In Nimmo WS, Tucker
        GT, eds: *Clinical Measurement in Drug Evaluation.* New York, John Wiley & Sons, Inc., 1995.

Chapter 14
1.   Bombardier C, Laine L, Reicin A, et al. Comparison of upper gastrointestinal toxicity of
        rofecoxib and naproxen in patients with rheumatoid arthritis. VIGOR Study Group. *N Engl J
        Med* 2000;343:1520-8.

2.   Bresalier RS, Sandler RS, Quan H, et al. Cardiovascular events associated with rofecoxib in a
        colorectal adenoma chemoprevention trial. *N Engl J Med* 2005;352:1092-102.

3.   Furberg CD, Levin AA, Gross PA, Shapiro RS, Strom BL. FDA and drug safety — a proposal
        for sweeping changes. *Arch Intern Med* 2006;166:1938-42

4.   Gunnell D, Ashby D. Antidepressants and suicide: what is the balance of benefit and harm. *Br
        Med J* 2004;329:34-8.

5.   Ioannidis JP, Lau J. Completeness of safety reporting in randomized trials: an evaluation of 7
        medical areas. *JAMA* 2001;285:437-43.

6. Kelly WN. Can the frequency and risks of fatal adverse drug events be determined? *Pharmacotherapy* 2001;21:521-7.

7. Lazarou J, Pomeranz BH, Corey PN. Incidence of adverse drug reactions in hospitalized patients: a meta-analysis of prospective studies. *JAMA* 1998;279:1200-5.

8. Pirmohamed M, James S, Green C, et al. Adverse drug reactions as cause of admission to hospital: prospective analysis of 18,820 patients. *Br Med J* 2004;329:15-9.

9. Silverstein FE, Faich G, Goldstein JL, et al. Gastrointestinal toxicity with celecoxib vs non-steroidal anti-inflammatory drugs for osteoarthritis and rheumatoid arthritis: the CLASS study: a randomized controlled trial. Celecoxib Long-term Arthritis Safety Study. *JAMA* 2000;284:1247-55.

10. Solomon S, McMurray JJV, Pfeffer MA, et al. Cardiovascular risk associated with celecoxib in clinical trial for colorectal adenoma prevention. *N Engl J Med* 2005;352:1071-80.

11. Strom BL. Potential for conflict of interest in the evaluation of suspected adverse drug reactions: a counterpoint. *JAMA* 2004;292:2643-6.

12. Wang PS, Bohn RL, Glynn RJ, et al. Hazardous benzodiazepine regimens in the elderly: effects of half-life, dosage, and duration on risk of hip fracture. *Am J Psychiatry* 2001;158:892-8.

Chapter 15
1. Furberg CD, Hawkins CM, Lichstein E, for the Beta-Blocker Heart Attack Trial Study Group. Effect of propranolol in postinfarction patients with mechanical or electrical complications. *Circulation* 1984;69:761-5.

2. Kaariainen I, Sipponen P, Siurala M. What fraction of hospital ulcer patients is eligible for prospective drug trials? *Scand J Gastroenterol* 1991;186:73-6.

3. Psaty BM, Rhoads C, Furberg CD. Evidence-based medicine. Worship of form and treatment of high blood pressure. *J Gen Intern Med* 2000;15:755-6.

4. Rochon PA, Berger PB, Gordon M. The evolution of clinical trials: inclusion and representation. *CMAJ* 1998;159:1373-4.

Chapter 16
1. Anturane Reinfarction Trial Research Group: Sulfinpyrazone in the prevention of sudden death after myocardial infarction. *N Engl J Med* 1980;302:250-6.

2. Coronary Drug Project Research Group. Influence of adherence to treatment and response of cholesterol on mortality in the Coronary Drug Project. *N Engl J Med* 1980;303:1038-41.

3. Granger BB, Swedberg K, Ekman I, et al. for the CHARM investigators. Adherence to candesartan and placebo and outcomes in chronic heart failure in the CHARM programme: double-blind, randomised, controlled clinical trial. *Lancet* 2005;366:2005-11.

4. Simpson SH, Eurich DT, Majumdar SR, et al. A meta-analysis of the association between adherence to drug therapy and mortality. *Br Med J*, 2006; 333:15; doi:10.1136/bmj.38875.675486.55.

5. Temple R, Pledger GW. The FDA's critique of the Anturane Reinfarction Trial. *N Engl J Med* 1980;303:1488-92.

Chapter 17
1. Carlberg B, Samuelsson O, Lindholm LH. Atenolol in hypertension: is it a wise choice? *Lancet* 2004;364:1684-9.

2.   Dahlöf B, Devereux RB, Kjeldsen SE, et al. Cardiovascular morbidity and mortality in the Losartan Intervention For Endpoint reduction in hypertension study (LIFE): a randomised trial against atenolol. *Lancet* 2002;359:995-1003.

3.   Dahlöf B, Sever PS, Poulter NR, et al. for the ASCOT investigators. Prevention of cardiovascular events with an antihypertensive regimen of amlodipine adding perindopril as required versus atenolol adding bendroflumethiazide as required, in the Anglo-Scandinavian Cardiac Outcomes Trial-Blood Pressure Lowering Arm (ASCOT-BPLA): a multicentre randomized controlled trial. *Lancet* 2005;366:895-906.

4.   Danish Omeprazole Study Group. Omeprazole and cimetidine in the treatment of ulcers of the body of the stomach: a double blind comparative trial. *Br Med J* 1989;298:645-7.

5.   Dormandy JA, Charbonnel B, Eckland DJA, et al. on behalf of the PROactive investigators. Secondary prevention of macrovascular events in patients with type 2 diabetes in the PROactive Study (PROspective pioglitAzone Clinical Trial in macroVascular Events): a randomized controlled trial. *Lancet* 2005;366:1279-89.

6.   Freemantle N, Cleland J, Young P, Mason J, Harrison J. β–blockade after myocardial infarction: systematic review and meta regression analysis. *Br Med J* 1999;318:1730-7.

7.   Francis CW, Berkowitz SD, Comp PC, et al. Comparison of ximelagatran with warfarin for the prevention of venous thromboembolism after total knee replacement. *N Engl J Med* 2003;349:1703-12.

8.   Heres S, Davis J, Maino K, et al. Why olanzapine beats risperidone, risperidone beats quetiapine, and quetiapine beats olanzapine: An exploratory analysis of head-to-head comparison studies of second-generation antipsychotics. *Am J Psychiatry* 2006;163:185-94.

9.   Johansen HK, Gøtzsche PC. Problems in the design and reporting of trials of antifungal agents encountered during meta-analysis. *JAMA* 1999;282:1752-9.

10.   Jørgensen KJ, Johansen HK, Gøtzsche PC. Flaws in design, analysis and interpretation of Pfizer's antifungal trials of voriconazole and uncritical subsequent quotations. *Trials* 2006;7:3.

11.   Kahrilas PJ, Falk GW, Johnson DA, et al. Esomeprazole improves healing and symptom resolution as compared with omeprazole in reflux oesophagitis patients: a randomized controlled trial. The Esomeprazole Study Investigators. *Aliment Pharmacol Ther* 2000;14:1249-58.

12.   Lindholm LH, Carlberg B, Samuelsson O. Should β-blockers remain first choice in the treatment of primary hypertension? A meta-analysis. *Lancet* 2005;366:1545-53.

13.   Poole-Wilson PA, Swedberg K, Cleland JG, et al. Comparison of carvedilol and metoprolol on clinical outcomes in patients with chronic heart failure in the Carvedilol Or Metoprolol European Trial (COMET): randomised controlled trial. *Lancet* 2003;362:7-13.

14.   Psaty BM, Lumley T, Furberg CD, et al. Health outcomes associated with various antihypertensive therapies used as first-line agents. A network meta-analysis. *JAMA* 2003;289:2534-44.

15.   Psaty BM, Weiss N, Furberg CD. Recent trials in hypertension. Compelling science or commercial speech? *JAMA* 2006;295:1704-6.

16.   Rochon PA, Gurwitz JH, Simms RW, et al. A study of manufacturer-supported trials of nonsteroidal anti-inflammatory drugs in the treatment of arthritis. *Arch Intern Med* 1994;154:157-63.

17.   Watson P, Stjernchantz J. A six-month, randomized, double-masked study comparing
       latanoprost with timolol in open-angle glaucoma and ocular hypertension. The Latanoprost
       Study Group. *Ophthalmology* 1996;103:126-37.

18.   World Medical Association Declaration of Helsinki. Ethical principles for medical research
       involving human subjects. *JAMA* 2000;284:3043-5.

Chapter 18
1.   Briel M, Schwartz GC, Thompson PL et al. Effects of early treatment with statins on short-term
       clinical outcomes in acute coronary syndromes. A meta-analysis of randomized controlled
       trials. *JAMA* 2006;295:2046-56.

2.   Dahlöf B, Deveveux RB, Kjeldsen SE, et al. Cardiovascular morbidity and mortality in the
       Losartan Intervention For Endpoint reduction in hypertension study (LIFE): a randomised trial
       against atenolol. *Lancet* 2002;359:995-1003.

3.   Dormandy JA, Charbonnel B, Eckland DJA, et al. on behalf of the PROactive investigators.
       Secondary prevention of macrovascular events in patients with type 2 diabetes in the
       PROactive Study (PROspective pioglitAzone Clinical Trial in macroVascular Events): a
       randomized controlled trial. *Lancet* 2005;366:1279-89.

4.   Freemantle N, Calvert M, Wood J, et al. Composite outcomes in randomized trials: greater
       precision but with greater uncertainty? *JAMA* 2003;289:2554-9.

5.   Schwartz GG, Olsson AG, Ezekowitz MD, et al. Effects of atorvastatin on early recurrent
       ischemic events in acute coronary syndromes. The MIRACL Study: a randomized controlled
       trial. *JAMA* 2001;285:1711-8.

Chapter 19
1.   Collins R, Peto R, Armitage J. The MRC/BHF Heart Protection Study: preliminary results. *Int J
       Clin Pract* 2002;56:53-6.

2.   Graham DJ, Staffa JA, Shatin D, et al. Incidence of hospitalized rhabdomyolysis in patients
       with lipid-lowering drugs. *JAMA* 2004;292:2585-90.

3.   PROGRESS Collaborative Group: Randomised trial of perindopril-based blood pressure-
       lowering regimen among 6105 individuals with previous stroke or transient ischaemic attack.
       Lancet 2001;358:1033-41.

4.   Psaty BM, Furberg CD, Ray WA, et al. Potential for conflict of interest in the evaluation of
       suspected adverse drug reactions: use of cerivastatin and risk of rhabdomyolysis. *JAMA*
       2004;292:2622-31.

5.   Robins SJ, Collins D, Wittes JT, et al. Relation of gemfibrozil treatment and lipid levels with
       major coronary events. VA-HIT: A randomized controlled trial. *JAMA* 2001;285:1585-91.

6.   Scandinavian Simvastatin Survival Study Group. Randomised trial of cholesterol lowering in
       4444 patients with coronary heart disease: the Scandinavian Simvastatin Survival Study (4S).
       Lancet 1994;344:1383-9.

Chapter 20
1.   Angell M, Utiger RD, Wood AJ. Disclosure of authors' conflicts of interest: a follow-up. *N Engl
       J Med* 2000;342:586-7.

2.   Barnes DE, Bero LA. Why review articles on the health effects of passive smoking reach
       different conclusions. *JAMA* 1998;279:1566-70.

3.   Cain DM, Loewenstein G, Moore DA. The dirt on coming clean: perverse effects of disclosing conflicts of interest. *J Legal Studies* 2005;34:1-25.

4.   Djulbegovic B, Lacevic M, Cantor A, et al. The uncertainty principle and industry-sponsored research. *Lancet* 2000;356:635-8.

5.   Chaudhry S, Schroter S, Smith R, Morris J. Does declaration of competing interests affect readers' perceptions? A randomised trial. *Br Med J* 2002;325:1391-2.

6.   Heres S, Davis J, Maino K, et al. Why olanzapine beats risperidone, risperidone beats quetiapine, and quetiapine beats olanzapine: An exploratory analysis of head-to-head comparison studies of second-generation antipsychotics. *Am J Psychiatry* 2006;163:185-94.

7.   Kjaergard LL, Als-Nielsen B. Association between competing interests and authors' conclusions: epidemiological study of randomised clinical trials published in the *BMJ*. Available online at http://bmj.com/cgi/content/full/325/7358/249#BIBL .

8.   Lexchin J, Bero LA, Djulbegovic B, Clark O. Pharmaceutical industry sponsorship and research outcome and quality: systematic review. *Br Med J* 2003;326:1167-70.

9.   Ridker PM, Torres J. Reported outcomes in major cardiovascular clinical trials funded by for-profit and not-for-profit organizations: 2000-2005. *JAMA* 2006;295:2270-4.

10.   Stelfox HT, Chua G, O'Rourke K, Detsky AS. Conflict of interest in the debate over calcium-channel antagonists. *N Engl J Med* 1998;338:101-6.

Chapter 21
1.   Chan A-W, Altman DG. Epidemiology and reporting of randomised trials published in PubMed journals. *Lancet* 2005;365:1159-62.

2.   Chan A-W, Altman DG. Identifying outcome reporting bias in randomised trials on PubMed: review of publications and survey of authors. *Br Med J* 2005;330:753-9

3.   Melander H, Ahlqvist-Rastad J, Meijer G, Beermann B. Evidence b(i)ased medicine-selective reporting from studies sponsored by pharmaceutical industry: review of studies in new drug applications. *Br Med J* 2003;326:1171-3.

4.   Mills EJ, Wu P, Gagnier J, Devereaux PJ. The quality of randomized trial reporting in leading medical journals since the revised CONSORT statement. *Contemp Clin Trials* 2005;26:480-7.

5.   O'Shea JC, Califf RM. International differences in cardiovascular clinical trials. *Am Heart J* 2001;141:866-74.

6.   Relman AS. Are we a filter or a sponge? *N Engl J Med* 1978;299:197.

7.   Rothstein H, Sutton A, Borenstein M (eds). *Publication Bias in Meta-analysis: Prevention, Assessment, and Adjustments*. London, John Wiley & Sons, Ltd., 2005.

8.   Vickers A, Goyal N, Harland R, Rees R. Do certain countries produce only positive results? A systematic review of controlled trials. *Controlled Clin Trials* 1998;19:159-66.

Chapter 22
1.   ISIS-2 (Second International Study of Infarct Survival) Collaborative Group. Randomized trial of intravenous streptokinase, oral aspirin, both or neither, among 17187 cases of suspected acute myocardial infarction: ISIS-2. *Lancet* 1988;ii:349-60.

2.   Oakes D, Moss AJ, Fleiss JL, et al. Use of compliance measures in an analysis of the effect of diltiazem on mortality and reinfarction after myocardial infarction. *J Am Stat Assoc* 1993;88:44-9.

3.   Peto R. Statistical aspects of cancer trials, In Halnan KE, ed: *Treatment of Cancer*. London, Chapman & Hall, 1982.

Chapter 23

1.   Furberg CD, Herrington DM, Psaty BM. Are drugs within a class interchangeable? *Lancet* 1999;354:1202-4.

2.   Furberg CD, Pitt B. Are all angiotensin-converting enzyme inhibitors interchangeable? *J Am Coll Cardiol* 2001;37:1456-60.

3.   Luzier AB, Forrest A, Adelman M, et al. Impact of angiotensin-converting enzyme inhibitor underdosing on rehospitalization rates in congestive heart failure. *Am J Cardiol* 1998;82:465-9.

4.   Pitt B, O'Neill B, Feldman R, et al. The QUinapril Ischemic Event Trial (QUIET): Evaluation of chronic ACE inhibitor therapy in patients with ischemic heart disease and preserved left ventricular function. *Am J Cardiol* 2001;87:1058-63.

5.   PROGRESS Collaborative Group: Randomised trial of perindopril-based blood pressure-lowering regimen among 6105 individuals with previous stroke or transient ischaemic attack. *Lancet* 2001;358:1033-41.

Chapter 24

1.   Bell CM, Urbach DR, Ray JG, et al. Bias in published cost effectiveness studies: systematic review. *Br Med J* 2006;332:699-703.

2.   Cranor CW, Bunting BA, Christensen DB. The Asheville Project: Long-term clinical and economic outcomes of a community pharmacy diabetes care program. *J Am Pharm Assoc* 2003;43:173-84.

3.   Friedberg M, Saffran B, Stinson TJ, et al. Evaluation of conflict of interest in economic analyses of new drugs used in oncology. *JAMA* 1999;282:1453-7.

4.   Hill SR, Mitchell AS, Henry DA. Problems with the interpretation of pharmacoeconomic analyses. A review of submissions to the Australian pharmaceutical benefits scheme. *JAMA* 2000;283:2116-21.

5.   Hillman AL, Eisenberg JM, Pauly MV, et al. Avoiding bias in the conduct and reporting of cost-effectiveness research sponsored by pharmaceutical companies. *N Engl J Med* 1991:324:1362-5.

6.   Kassirer JP, Angell M. The journal's policy on cost-effectiveness analyses. *N Engl J Med* 1994;331:669-70.

7.   Paterson ML. Cost-benefit evaluation of a new technology for treatment of peptic ulcer disease. *Manage Decis Econ* 1983;4:50-62.

Chapter 25

1.   Djulbegovic B. Lifting the fog of uncertainty from the practice of medicine. *Br Med J* 2004;329:1419-20.

2.   Guyatt GH, Sackett DL, Cook DJ. Users' Guides to the Medical Literature: II. How to use an article about therapy or prevention: A. Are the results of the study valid? *JAMA* 1993;270:2598-601.

3.   Guyatt GH, Rennie D. *Users' Guides to the Medical Literature: Essentials of Evidence-Based Clinical Practice.* Chicago, IL, AMA Press, 2002.

Chapter 26
1.   Collins R, Julian D. British Hearth Foundation surveys (1987 and 1989) of United Kingdom treatment policies for acute myocardial infarction. *Br Heart J* 1991;66:250-5.

2.   Friedman L, Wenger NK, Knatterud GL. Impact of the Coronary Drug Project findings on clinical practice. *Controlled Clin Trials* 1983;4:513-22.

3.   Furberg RD, Furberg CD. Evaluating professional performance in cardiovascular medicine. *Evid Based Cardiovas Med* 2006;10:75-8.

4.   Grol R, Grimshaw J. From best evidence to best practice: effective implementation of change in patients' care. *Lancet* 2003;362:1225-30.

5.   Hyman DJ, Pavlik VN. Self-reported hypertension treatment practices among primary care physicians. Blood pressure thresholds, drug choices, and the role of guidelines and evidence-based medicine. *Arch Intern Med* 2000;160:2281-6.

6.   Lamas GA, Pfeffer MA, Hamm P, et al. Do the results of randomized clinical trials of cardiovascular drugs influence medical practice? *N Engl J Med* 1992;327:241-7.

7.   McGlynn EA, Asch SM, Adams J, et al. The quality of health care delivered to adults in the United States. *N Engl J Med* 2003;348:2635-45.

8.   Reiffel JA, Cook JR. Physician attitudes toward the use of type IC antiarrhythmics after the Cardiac Arrhythmia Suppression Trial (CAST). *Am J Cardiol* 1990;66:1262-4.

9.   Williams SC, Schmaltz SP, Morton DJ, et al. Quality of care in US hospitals as reflected by standardized measures, 2002-2004. *N Engl J Med* 2005;353:265-74.

Index

A

a priori, 39-43, 111
ACE inhibitor, 19, 21, 58, 69, 116
active control trials, 83-88
adherence, 80
adverse drug reactions, 67-71
adverse events
    late, 18
    rare, 17
    reporting, 70
    severity, 67-68
    unexpected, 19-20
albumin solutions, 27
ALLHAT, 96
analysis by treatment administered, 81
angiotensin receptor blocker (ARB), 21, 90
antiarrhythmics, 62, 69, 133
antibiotics, 109, 118
antifungal drug, 85-86
antipsychotics, 83-84, 101
Anturane Reinfarction Trial (ART), 79
ASCOT, 84
authorship, 99-102

B

barriers to optimal care, 133
benefit to harm balance, 2, 5-10, 91
beta-blocker, 75, 86, 117
bias
    ascertainment, 15
    indication, 35
    publication, 24, 104-106
    recall, 35
    selection, 35, 75
    sponsor, 88, 123
biologic markers, 61-65, 95-98
biostatistician, 107-113
blinded observer, 52
blinding/masking, 11, 15-16, 49-52

C

calcium channel blockers, 75, 100-101, 111, 117
Captopril Prevention Project, 47

Cardiac Arrhythmia Suppression Trial
    (CAST), 62, 69
case reports, 29, 30-31, 36
case series, 29, 31, 36
case-control studies, 29, 31-32, 36
causation, 68-70
chance finding, 109
checklist, 129
CLASS, 70-71
class effect, 115-119
clinical care, 131-135
ClinicalTrials.gov, 42
clinical trial
    definition, 11
    ethical limitations, 21-22
    strengths, 11-16
    weaknesses, 17-22
Cochrane Collaboration, 3, 126
cohort studies, 29, 33, 37
COMET, 86
compensatory treatment, 49
compliance, 7
composite outcomes, 89-93
confidence interval, 112-113
conflict-of-interest, 99
congenital abnormality, 30
control group, 13-14
Coronary Drug Project (CDP), 80, 132
corticosteroids, 26-27
cost-effectiveness, 122-124
COX-2 inhibitor, 70, 75, 118
CRASH, 27
critical appraisal, 2, 128
cross-sectional studies, 29, 31, 36

D

Declaration of Helsinki, 21
disease registries, 33
double-blind, 49

E

ecologic problems, 9
economic analysis, 121-124

About the Authors

Bengt D. Furberg, M.D., Ph.D. is Associate Professor of Clinical Physiology at the University of Uppsala, Sweden and is board-certified in internal medicine. He practiced medicine for 20 years and conducted several clinical trials in different indications. After spending a decade as medical director in the pharmaceutical industry, he serves as a medical consultant, evaluating the safety and efficacy of pharmaceutical products and medical devices and in the promotion of evidence-based medicine.

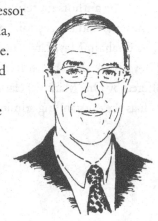

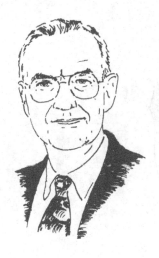

His brother, Curt D. Furberg, M.D., Ph.D., is Professor in the Division of Public Health Sciences, Wake Forest University School of Medicine, Winston-Salem, NC, USA. He received his medical training in Sweden. After arriving in the United States, he worked at the National Heart, Lung, and Blood Institute of the National Institutes of Health for 12 years. During this period, he was Head of the Clinical Trials Branch. His areas of interest are clinical trials, evidence-based medicine and drug safety. Dr. Furberg is co-author of the texts "Fundamentals of Clinical Trials"[1] and "Data Monitoring in Clinical Trials. A Case Studies Approach".[2]

The authors have acquired much of their knowledge about clinical studies through the "trial and error" method. Thus, they have personal experience about many of the problems they describe.

The authors gratefully acknowledge their colleagues' many valuable comments and suggestions on this text and its previous edition, in particular, Drs. Graham May, Lawrence Friedman, Bruce Psaty and Ms. Susan Margitić. They also wish to recognize the constructive suggestions on select chapters offered by Drs. Mark Espeland and Michelle Naughton, and Ms. Lynne Fox as well as the outstanding administrative support of Ms. Sarah Hutchens.

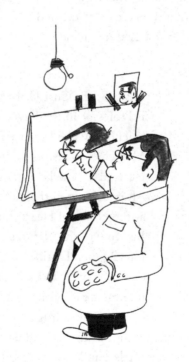

Cartoons by Nils Simonson, M.D.
Östersund, Sweden

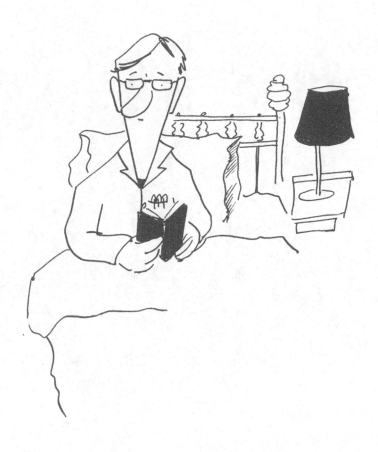

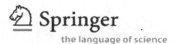
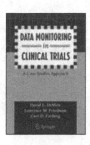

Data Monitoring in Clinical Trials: A Case Study Approach

David L. DeMets, Curt D. Furberg, and Lawrence M. Friedman (Editors)

Randomized clinical trials are the gold standard for establishing many clinical practice guidelines and are central to evidence based medicine. Obtaining the best evidence through clinical trials must be done within the boundaries of rigorous science and ethical principles. This book, through a series of case studies presented by many distinguished clinical trial experts, illustrates the complexity of this monitoring process. The editors provide an overview of the process and a summary of a multitude of the lessons learned from the cases presented.

2006. 374 p. Softcover ISBN 0-387-20330-0

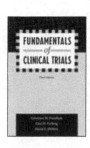

Fundamentals of Clinical Trials
Third Edition

Lawrence M. Friedman, Curt D. Furberg, and David L. DeMets

This text is structured to address the fundamentals as the protocol for a clinical trial is being developed. A chapter is devoted to each of the critical areas of a protocol to aid the clinical trial researcher. The fundamentals described in this text are based on sound scientific methodology, statistical principles and years of accumulated experience by the three authors. Collectively, the authors have been active researchers in a broad area of clinical trials including cardiology, cancer, ophthalmology, diabetes, osteoporosis, AIDS, women's health and screening tests. In these studies, the authors have served as members of the steering committee responsible for developing the protocol and as members of data and safety monitoring committees. The fundamentals were proposed in the first edition published in 1981 and have not changed substantially in the later editions. However, the number of examples illustrating the fundamentals has greatly expanded base on the collective experience of the authors.

1998. 361 pp. Softcover ISBN 978-0-387-98586-2